Dietary Supplements - Challenges and Future Research

Edited by A. Venketeshwer Rao and Leticia Rao

Published in London, United Kingdom

Dietary Supplements - Challenges and Future Research
http://dx.doi.org/10.5772/intechopen.95717
Edited by A. Venketeshwer Rao and Leticia Rao

Contributors
Maja Ergović Ravančić, Valentina Obradović, Paschal Chukwudi Aguihe, Ibinabo Imuetinyan Ilaboya, Deji Abiodun Joshua, Abdul Hei, Laishram Sanahanbi, Simon Welham, Lisa Coneyworth, Elizabeth Eveleigh, A. Venketeshwer Rao, Leticia Rao

First published in London, United Kingdom, 2023 by IntechOpen
IntechOpen is the global imprint of INTECHOPEN LIMITED, registered in England and Wales, registration number: 11086078, 5 Princes Gate Court, London, SW7 2QJ, United Kingdom

British Library Cataloguing-in-Publication Data
A catalogue record for this book is available from the British Library

Additional hard and PDF copies can be obtained from orders@intechopen.com

Dietary Supplements - Challenges and Future Research
Edited by A. Venketeshwer Rao and Leticia Rao
p. cm.
Print ISBN 978-1-80356-206-3
Online ISBN 978-1-80356-207-0
eBook (PDF) ISBN 978-1-80356-208-7

Meet the editors

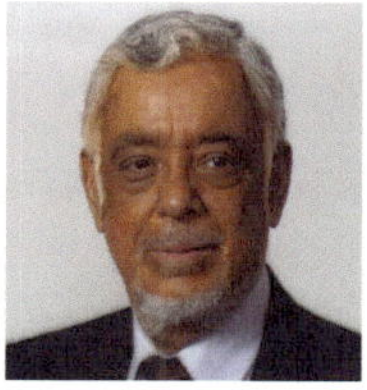

Dr. Rao is a Professor Emeritus in the Department of Nutritional Sciences, Faculty of Medicine, University of Toronto, Ontario, Canada. He is an expert in diet and health and his research has focused on the role of oxidative stress and antioxidant phytochemicals in the causation and prevention of chronic diseases, with emphasis on the role of carotenoids and polyphenols. His research interests also include the role of prebiotics and probiotics in human health. He has 100 publications in scientific journals and several books and book chapters to his credit. Dr. Rao has had a distinguished academic career spanning more than 45 years. He is popularly sought after by the international media for his opinions about nutrition and health.

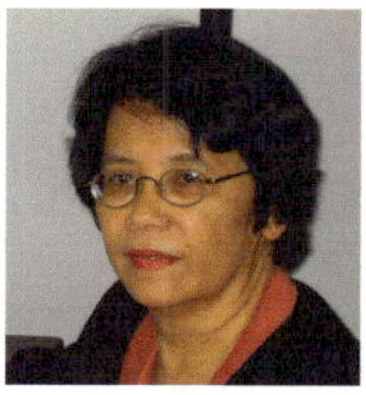

Dr. Leticia Rao is a Professor Emeritus at the University of Toronto, Ontario, Canada, and former director of the Calcium Research Laboratory at the same university. She is also a former staff scientist at St. Michael's Hospital, Toronto, Ontario. Her expertise is in bone cell biology with a focus on preventing osteoporosis. She studies bone cells in the laboratory and carries out basic and clinical studies of drugs, nutritional supplements, and phytonutrients including carotenoids and polyphenols in postmenopausal women. Her research has been presented at national and international conferences and symposia and she has published extensively in peer-reviewed scientific journals. She has co-authored one book and edited eight others on nutrition and health. Dr. Rao has frequently presented her work at international organisations.

Contents

Preface

Dietary supplements, also referred to as phytonutrients, nutraceuticals, and functional ingredients, contain not only essential vitamins and minerals but also beneficial compounds present in the diet. Recently, there has been a great deal of interest from consumers, health professionals, and regulatory agencies in the use, benefits, safety, and regulatory guidelines of dietary supplements. Unlike vitamins and minerals, phytonutrients do not have recommended levels of daily intake; rather, consumers are advised to consume foods that are good sources of these phytonutrients as part of a healthy diet. Manufacturers of health supplements have taken advantage of the surging interest in these products, claiming that they play an important role in the management of health. The overall interest in supplements has also prompted health professionals to undertake extensive research and develop guidelines for their consumption and safety. Regulatory agencies are also working to make sure that supplements are safe and meet manufacturers' health claims.

In recognition of the new information on the composition of dietary supplements, the health issues they are claimed to be beneficial for, their mechanisms of action, and safe levels of consumption, *Dietary Supplements - Challenges and Future Research* provides readers with information to better understand the positive and negative outcomes of consuming supplements. This book contains chapters written by international researchers that address some important aspects of dietary supplements. It is organized into three sections.

Section 1, "An Overview of the Role of Dietary Supplements in Human Health," includes one chapter. Chapter 1 by Rao and Rao called " Introductory Chapter: Dietary Supplements, Definitions, Role in Human Health and Regulatory Issues" is an introduction to the need for and the role of dietary supplements in the management of health and prevention of diseases. It defines dietary supplements, presents recent research findings, and discusses regulatory guideline issues. It concludes by identifying the challenges facing these products and the need for further research for a better understanding of the role supplements play in human health.

Section 2 "Dietary Supplements in Health Management" includes three chapters. Chapter 2, "Supplements and Down Syndrome" by Maja Ergović Ravančić and Valentina Obradović, Chapter 3 "Impact of Glycine Supplementation to Dietary Crude Protein Reduction in Broiler Chickens," by Paschal Chukwudi Aguihe et al., and Chapter 4, "DHA (Docosahexaenoic Acid): A Biomolecule with Diverse Roles and Health Benefits" by Abdul Hei and Laishram Sanahanbi. Together, these three chapters address the role of dietary supplements in disease and health management using human and animal studies.

Section 3 "Dietary Sources" includes one chapter. Chapter 5, "The Role of Micronutrients and Micronutrient Supplements in Vegetarian and Vegan Diets" by Elizabeth Eveleigh,

Lisa Coneyworth and Simon Welham presents information on the presence of micronutrients in vegetarian and vegan diets and discusses the significance of these diets in meeting the recommended levels of nutrients.

Overall, this book provides important information to consumers, health professionals, researchers, and regulatory agencies that are helpful for understanding various aspects of dietary supplements as well as the challenges faced in human health. It also provides a guide to future research in the field.

A. Venketeshwer Rao
Professor Emeritus,
Faculty of Medicine,
Department of Nutritional Sciences,
University of Toronto,
Ontario, Canada

Leticia Rao
Professor Emeritus,
University of Toronto,
Toronto, Canada

Section 1

An Overview of the Role of Dietary Supplements in Human Health

Chapter 1

Introductory Chapter: Dietary Supplements, Definitions, Role in Human Health and Regulatory Issues

A. Venketeshwer Rao and Leticia Rao

1. Introduction

National dietary guidelines are the ideal way to meet all the nutritional requirements for a healthy life. However for genetic, health or lifestyle-related activities, not everyone can follow these dietary guidelines. Not following the dietary guidelines can result in individuals not being able to meet their nutritional requirements leading to health-related issues. In the belief that they may not be meeting the required levels of nutrients, either justified or not, they take 'supplements' as insurance towards nutrient adequacy and good health. A common understanding of dietary supplements is presented in **Table 1**. **Figure 1** shows a typical dietary supplement fact of a commercial product [1]. Traditionally, the focus of dietary supplements is essential vitamins and minerals. However, in recent years, other biologically active components of foods have also been identified as playing an important role in human health [2, 3]. Although technically they are not 'nutrients', they are referred to as 'phytonutrients', 'nutraceuticals', functional ingredients' and 'bioactive beneficial compounds. They include compounds such as carotenoids, polyphenols, dietary fibre and many more from plant and animal kingdoms. Nutritionists and other health professionals now believe that consuming these phytonutrients as part of a

- A dietary supplement is a product that is manufactured with the aim of supplementing one's regular diet. They are not intended to treat, diagnose, prevent or cure diseases.
- They are either natural compounds extracted from food sources or synthetic.
- Traditionally they include vitamins and minerals in the form of multivitamin and mineral preparations.
- May also contain fibre, amino acids and fatty acids.
- May also contain other nonessential substances claimed to have beneficial health effects such as plant pigments, polyphenols and other biologically active compounds, including animal-derived compounds.
- May also contain animal-derived compounds such as collagen.
- They may be marketed individually or as a combination.
- They often contain health claims such as supporting heart, brain, eye health and bone strength.

Table 1.
Understanding what a dietary supplement is.

Suggested use: As a dietary supplement, take two (2) gummy vitamins per day. Chew thoroughly before swallowing.

Supplement Facts

Serving Size 2 Gummy Vitamins

Amount Per Serving		**% Daily Value for Pregnant & Lactating Women**	**Amount Per Serving**		**% Daily Value for Pregnant & Lactating Women**
Calories	20		Folic acid	800 mcg	100%
Total Carbohydrate	4 g	**	Vitamin B-12 (as cyanocobalamin)	8 mcg	100%
Sugars	3 g	**	Zinc (as zinc chelate)	3.8 mg	25%
Vitamin A (as retinyl palmitate)	4000 IU	50%	Choline (as choline chloride)	10 mg	**
Vitamin C (as ascorbic acid)	30 mg	50%	Omega-3 fatty acids (from fish oil)	65 mg	**
Vitamin D (as cholecalciferol)	400 IU	100%	DHA (Docosahexaenoic acid)	50 mg	**
Vitamin E (as d-alpha-tccopheryl acetate)	15 IU	50%	Other Omega-3 fatty acids	15 mg	**
Niacin (as incsitol niacinate)	20 mg	100%			
Vitamin B-6 (as pyridoxine HCl)	2.5 mg	100%			

** Daily Value not established.

Other ingredients: Glucose syrup, sucrose, water, gelatin; less than 2% of: citric acid, colors (blueberry and carrot concentrates, purple carrot juice concentrate), fumaric acid, lactic acid, and natural flavors. **Contains: fish (tuna).**

This product uses high quality, purified fish oil that has been tested for mercury and PCBs.

Figure 1.
Typical dietary supplement facts of a commercial product [1].

daily diet is beneficial to maintain good health and avoiding diseases. However, being a new area of research, in most cases, there are no recommended levels of their intake except to advise consumers to include foods that are good sources of these phytonutrients as part of their healthy diet. This concept of taking supplements has gained popularity in recent years. Recognising the potential for a business opportunity, business sectors around the globe are now offering a wide range of dietary and nutritional supplements. This increase in the intake and sales of supplements has raised serious concerns among health professionals and government regulatory agencies. Questions are now being raised regarding the validity of the scientific evidence in support of supplements and possible misuse leading to adverse effects. In view of the importance of the issue of dietary supplements, several review articles have been published over the years [4–8], and it was felt that there was a need for a book on this topic to provide current knowledge on the research that is being conducted and provide science-based opinions relating to the use of supplements.

2. Challenges and future research

Undoubtedly, nutrient deficiencies such as vitamin A, iron, folic acid and vitamin D, to name a few, have been documented to affect the health of infants, children and childbearing women in the developing parts of the world. However, they are not restricted only to developing countries but also to industrialised countries. The reasons could include genetic factors, insufficient access to proper food, insufficient knowledge of nutrient requirements and their sources, and lifestyle factors. Dietary supplements, therefore, have a rightful place in providing the needed nutrients and other beneficial bioactive compounds to at-risk needy consumers. As a result, sales of these supplements have increased globally, indicating the awareness of the need for these compounds to maintain good health. However, there are still many challenges that the scientific community, consumers, manufacturers and regulatory agencies face in ensuring that the supplements being marketed and consumed are safe and indeed provide the healthy benefits claimed on the label [5].

As more and more new information is available relating to dietary supplements, one of the first challenges facing consumers and regulatory agencies is to define and understand what a dietary supplement is and differentiate them from medicines. Two important aspects of being considered are the intended use of the product and the claim(s) the product is associated with [6, 8]. In countries like the USA, Canada and

Australia, dietary supplements are considered as being self-selecting with limited claims in support of overall health and wellness and not requiring a prescription from a medical practitioner [5]. However, these guidelines are not always universally applied and vary from country to country. As mentioned in their article by Dwyer et al. [5], melatonin is regulated in the USA as a dietary supplement, in Canada as a Natural Health Product (NHP), and in Australia as a prescription medicine. As more and more marketing of dietary supplements is becoming a global issue, a clear and well-defined definition is essential to minimise confusion.

Another challenge is to have good science-based evidence in support of the claims that are often associated with dietary supplements. The two considerations that are important relate to the compound itself that is being evaluated and the design of the study being used. With respect to the compound itself, its source, purity and scientifically valid analytical procedures for its evaluation are important. With regard to the study design, if is absolutely essential that it is in accordance with scientifically accepted procedures of being double-blind with appropriate controls. If it is a clinical trial, the nature of the subjects participating, their health status, gender and age, length of administration of the compound being administered, procedures used to evaluate end results, and statistical procedures used in arriving at the results. In other words, the results derived from the study followed all the scientifically accepted procedures.

In addition to the challenges mentioned above, one of the most important challenges is faced by the regulatory agencies [5]. Unfortunately, no one regulatory model is used globally based on their regional priorities and needs. However, one common consideration of the different regulatory models used globally is to assure the consumers that the dietary supplements are safe and meet the claims made by the manufacturers. We have come a long way in developing a regulatory framework to achieve the goals of safety and applicability. However, as more and more new compounds are now being identified as beneficial for good health and marketing, much more work needs to be done in the future.

This introductory chapter aims to provide readers with a better understanding of the need for dietary supplements, what they are and the challenges faced by the industry, consumers, scientists and regulatory agencies. The common goal of all these stakeholders is safety and good health.

Author details

A. Venketeshwer Rao* and Leticia Rao
University of Toronto, Toronto, Ontario, Canada

*Address all correspondence to: venket.rao18@gmail.com

References

[1] Available from: https://www.mouseprint.org/2014/09/01/some-online-stores-make-shoppers-buy-vitamins-blindly/

[2] Rao V. Phytochemicals. A Global Perspective of their Role in Nutrition and Health. London, UK: IntechOpen; 2012

[3] Rao AV, Manns D, Rao L, editors. Phytochemical in Human Health. London, UK: IntechOpen; 2020

[4] Abubakar AA et al. A review on dietary supplements: Health benefits, market trends, and challenges. 2020. International Journal of Scientific Development and Research. 2020;**5**:26-34

[5] Dwyer JT, Coates PM, Smith MJ. Dietary supplements: Regulatory challenges and research resources. Nutrients. 2018;**10**:41-64

[6] Coates PM, Betz JM, Blackman MR, Crogg GM, Levine M, Moss J, et al., editors. Encyclopedia of Nutritional Supplements. 2nd ed. Boca Raton: CRC Press; 2010

[7] Journal of Dietary supplements. Taylor and Francis. Available from: https://www.tandforline.com/journals/ijds20

[8] US Food & Drug Administration. What's New in Dietary Supplements. Washington DC: US Food & Drug Administration; 2022

Section 2

Dietary Supplements in Health Management

Chapter 2

Supplements and Down Syndrome

Maja Ergović Ravančić and Valentina Obradović

Abstract

Down syndrome (DS) is one of the most common genetic disorders associated with a number of difficulties that are visible through the motor and cognitive development. Some theories claim that intake of supplements in very high doses could upgrade the physical and intellectual status of individuals with DS. Numerous papers have been published to support these theories, but at the same time, a great number of papers have warned of the risks of uncontrolled, excessive use of dietary supplements and asked for the proof of such claims by independent scientific studies. In this chapter, we will provide a review of the most commonly used supplements and major findings on this matter. Open access to information about the positive and negative sides of such supplementation is primarily important for guardians of people with DS in order to make the decision whether to use such preparations. It could also be an incentive for scientists to focus on the development of beneficial and safe therapies.

Keywords: Down syndrome, trisomy 21, oxidative stress, supplements, genes

1. Introduction

The aim of this chapter is to provide the reader with scientifically based information about the possibilities and dangers of using nutritional supplements for individuals with Down syndrome (DS). DS or trisomy 21, first described by Dr. John Langdon Down in 1866, is one of the most common genetic disorders that impact fetal development. It is a chromosomal disorder where an individual has an additional copy of chromosome 21, which may be full or partial [1]. The prevalence of children with DS worldwide is between 1:319 and 1:1000, and depends on the age of the mother (1/2000 in teenage girls to 1/40 in 42-year-old women) sociocultural, religious variables, and the possibility of terminating a pregnancy [2–4]. Every child with DS has unique phenotypic characteristics on which their overall physical and cognitive development depends, so the medical conditions associated with DS are not the same for every child (**Figure 1**). Considering the high cure rate of various comorbidities from which a DS child can suffer before and after birth, the mortality rate fell from 14.2% to 2.3% [5]. The life expectancy of people with DS has increased significantly over the last century, up to 60 years [6]. The use of nutritional supplements for children with DS is a topic that is extremely important for parents and caregivers as they want to improve their child's cognitive functions and health. However, the danger to the child can arise when the use of dietary supplements is uncontrolled, in large doses, and without a prior nutritional status of the organism. The program of early intervention with dietary supplements has been increasingly mentioned in connection with DS,

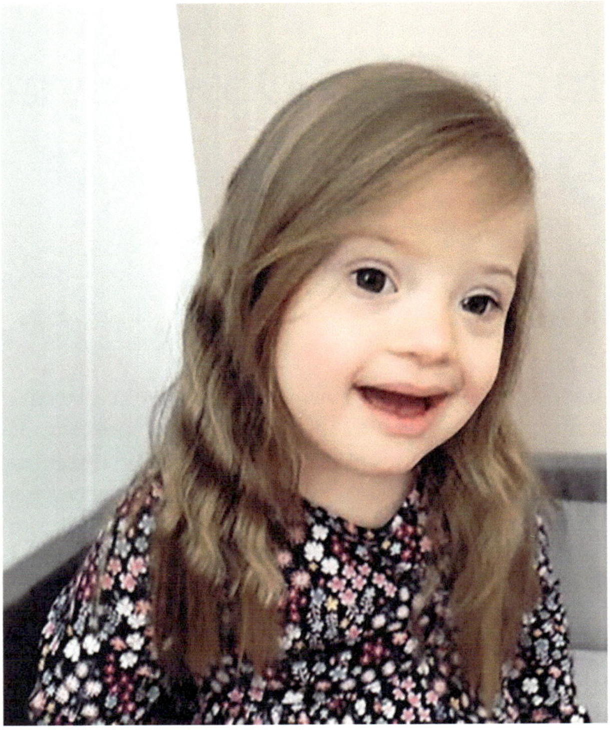

Figure 1.
A three-year-old child with Down syndrome. (source: author).

however, research on the benefits of their use is still very unsupported by concrete evidence that would give doctors guidance for their recommendation.

2. Down syndrome

Since the discovery that DS is a result of trisomy 21, the main interest of the studies has been the identification of human chromosome 21 genes (Hsa21), and the impact of their overexpression on the DS phenotype [7]. To explain the similarities and differences in the phenotypic characteristics associated with DS, a gene dose imbalance theory has been hypothesized stating that patients with DS have an increased dose or number of gene copies on Hsa21, which may lead to increased gene expression. This includes the possibility that specific genes or subsets of genes can control specific phenotypes of DS, but also that a nonspecific dose of a number of trisomic genes leads to a genetic imbalance that has a major impact on the expression and regulation of many other genes throughout the genome. Phenotypic analyzes found that only one or a few small chromosomal regions, termed "critical regions of Down syndrome," (DSCR) a region of 3.8–6.5 Mb at 21q21.22, with approximately 30 genes are responsible for most DS phenotypes [8, 9]. There are numerous physical features and congenital conditions specific to DS, resulting from overexpression of genes caused by the extra chromosome presented in **Table 1**. Every child is unique and features and conditions are not equally expressed and represented.

Physical features	
Head	Small, shortened skull that is flattened on the back, sloping forehead, missing or underdeveloped sinuses.
Eyes	Upward slanted and wide-set eyes, brushfield spots, and epicanthal folds.
Ears	Ears set lower on the head and smaller ears with extra folds.
Nose	Smaller nose and flattened nasal bridge.
Mouth	Smaller mouth, large tongue that tends to stick out more often, undersized teeth, crooked teeth, and irregularly shaped teeth.
Hands	Short fingers, broad hands, only one crease across the palm, and curved fifth finger.
Feet	Larger gap between the first and the second toe.
Limbs	Short and stocky arms and legs with hyperflexible joints.
Body	Short stature, shorter and wider neck, protruding stomach.
Congenital condition	
Heart	Septal defects (atrial septal defect, ventricular septal defect, and atrioventricular septal defect), patent ductus arteriosus, and tetralogy of Fallot.
Vision	Glaucoma, refractive errors, cataracts, amblyopia, and blepharitis.
Hearing	Hearing loss (conductive and sensorineural), glue ear, and otitis media.
Musculoskeletal	Hypotonia, ligamentous laxity, atlantoaxial instability, hip abnormalities, kneecap instability, and flat feet.
Digestive	Hirschsprung disease, tracheoesophageal fistula, duodenal atresia, esophageal atresia, imperforate anus, and gastroesophageal reflux disorder.
Immune	Hypothyroidism, respiratory infections, and celiac disease.

Table 1.
Possible physical features and congenital conditions associated with Down syndrome [9].

Promoting the health of people with DS is extremely important because it creates a prerequisite for improving their quality of life. Dietary composition, macronutrient and micronutrient intake, eating habits, and lifestyle can be fundamental for maintaining good health. Proper nutrition can have a major impact on preventing or delaying the onset of certain diseases in people with DS. However, very often nutrients from food are not enough to fulfill the daily needs for basic nutrients due to difficulties with swallowing and chewing, excessive sensory sensitivity, and numerous health problems, such as celiac disease. Cardiopathy in infants can impair food tolerance and adverse conditions may increase the frequency of aspiration [10].

In order to compensate for the lack of key nutrients necessary for the proper functioning of the body and fill the gap between diet and health in children with DS, dietary supplements can be used, but their usage should be controlled and in accordance with the identified deficiencies in the body.

3. History of nutritional supplementation for DS

Based on the assumption that an extra chromosome causes a metabolic imbalance that can be affected by various dietary supplements, Dr. Henry Turkel developed the first formulation composed of 48 different substances called "U-series" in the 1940s. The Food and Drug Administration (FDA) rejected his request for a new drug because it could not serve as a cure. A modified supplement formula was developed by Dr. Jack Warner during the 1980s as high-performance capsules (HAP Caps), which contained high doses of dietary antioxidants, such as vitamins A, E, and C, digestive enzymes, minerals zinc (Zn), copper (Cu), manganese (Mn), and selenium (Se), in order to correct metabolic disorders. HAP caps were formulated in the FDA laboratory and had approval from 1986 until his death in 2004 [11, 12]. During this period, Dixie Lawrence Tafoya, combining elements of both treatments with the addition of new ingredients, developed a combination of targeted nutritional intervention (TNI) supplements that included amino acids and smart drugs (Piracetam) in addition to various micronutrients. These supplements were promoted under the name Nutrivene. In Canada, under the leadership of Kent Macleod, Nutrichem Laboratories has launched a supplement called "MSB Plus" in accordance with the standards of good manufacturing practice at the licensed Health Canada Site. Despite the fact that various supplements have been applied to children with DS since the 1950s, repeated studies have shown that there are no nutritional deficiencies that would apply to all children with DS. Furthermore, there is no objective study that has confirmed the need for any of these supplements, with the possible exception of the minerals Zn and Se [12, 13].

Sacks & Buckley [12] pointed out the lack of well-designed scientific studies and warned of the danger of overdose in the case of supplement introduction in addition to a balanced diet. Many studies that support supplementation involved a small number of subjects, a wide range of age participants, short duration, and very few randomized controlled and blind studies [14, 15].

The popularity of supplements was confirmed by a survey among 1,200 respondents in the US, Brazil, and the EU that found that almost half of pediatric patients with DS have used or are currently using dietary supplements. 20% of surveyed parents who gave their child supplements haven't informed the pediatrician about it. Above all, supplements given to children with DS often exceeded the recommended daily doses [16]. Nevertheless, dietary supplements for DS still receive a lot of attention from parents, which leads to efforts of scientists to define the possible benefits of dietary supplements for people with DS-based on scientifically based knowledge.

4. DS issues targeted by nutritional supplementation

4.1 Oxidative stress

The theory of oxidative stress involves the occurrence of oxygen radicals, called reactive oxygen species (ROS) during oxidative metabolism. ROS include superoxides ($O_2 \bullet^-$) and hydroxyl ($OH \bullet$) free radicals and other molecules, such as hydrogen peroxide (H_2O_2) and peroxynitrite which have the ability to become very harmful to cells. To defend against ROS, cells developed various mechanisms to eliminate them: antioxidant enzymes (superoxide dismutase (SOD), glutathione peroxidase (GPx), and catalase (CAT)) along with antioxidants, such as vitamins C, E, or glutathione. If an imbalance between oxidants and antioxidants happens in cells, oxidative stress occurs [17, 18]. Numerous studies point to oxidative stress as a possible explanation for a number of DS-related problems, such as intellectual disability, accelerated aging, and cognitive and neuronal dysfunction [14, 19–21].

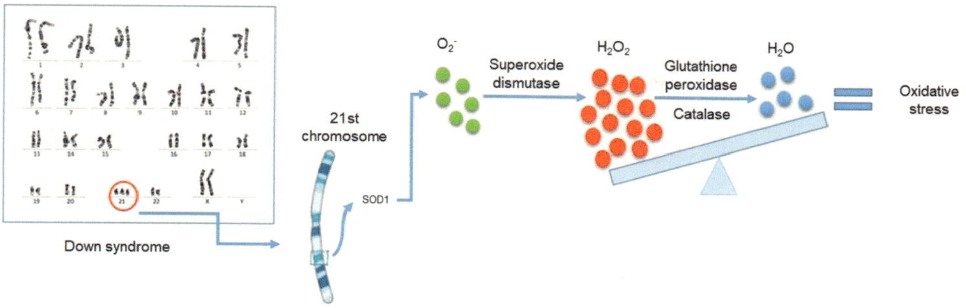

Figure 2.
Oxidative stress in Down syndrome.

The 21st chromosome contains SOD1 gene, which encodes the enzyme Cu-Zn superoxide dismutase (Cu-Zn SOD), responsible for the conversion of O_2^- to H_2O_2 in the cytosol. Increased SOD1 activity results in the creation of elevated levels of H_2O_2 that should be effectively removed by other enzymes, such as CAT, GPx, and thioredoxin peroxidase. Excess of chromosomes leads to overexpression of the SOD1 gene, and to elevated H_2O_2 levels that cannot be completely eliminated by CAT and GPx, so overproduction of ROS occurs (**Figure 2**) [22–25]. SOD1 was found to be 50% higher than normal in various cells and tissues of people with DS, so the SOD1/GPx activity ratio was consequently altered [19, 22, 26–29].

Strydom et al. [30] in his study on 32 adults with DS could not confirm the hypothesis that an increased SOD1/GPx ratio leads to low cognitive results. Surprisingly, they found that a low SOD1/GPx ratio leads to bad memory ability. They also pointed out that other possible factors could also affect SOD1 and GPx activity, such as regular exercise, Se, and homocysteine levels.

4.2 Cognitive development

Research has shown that the maturation of certain areas of the brain during childhood is associated with the development of specific cognitive functions, such as language, reading, and memory [31, 32]. Rapid brain growth occurs during the first 2 years of life (at age 2, the brain reaches 80% of an adult's weight), so this period of life may be particularly sensitive to nutritional deficiencies [33].

Nutrition, as the link between nutrients and health, should provide the building blocks needed to build and maintain the structure and function of the central nervous system. The intellectual disorder occurs when a child fails to fully develop the intellectual ability to think, reason, learn and understand. Children with intellectual disabilities also have problems in learning adaptive behavior, which encompasses the social and practical skills needed for everyday life. Intellectual impairment varies among children with Down syndrome. It ranges from a severe intellectual impairment that makes people completely dependent on caregivers, to mild effects that allow people to think and learn at levels that allow them to continue their higher education, keep their jobs, and live independently.

It is thought that nutrition may play a key role in brain development, and, thus intellectual functioning. The brain, similar to the rest of the body, needs proteins, fats, carbohydrates, vitamins, and minerals to grow and function, which are ingested through food or supplementation if food intake is difficult. As the brain develops faster than the rest of the body, it is obvious to consider that a lack of nutrition at a critical stage of development can lead to permanent changes in the structure and functioning of the brain. In addition, the brain is the most metabolically active organ in the body, but it has very limited energy reserves, so it relies on a diet for a continuous supply of glucose. Similarly, minute-by-minute brain function requires an adequate supply of micronutrients that act as coenzymes or form structural parts of enzymes required for optimal metabolic activity [34, 35].

4.3 Neurodegenerative diseases

Since individuals with DS are prone to elevated levels of oxidative stress at an early age and consequent accumulation of ROS, which are cytotoxic byproducts of normal mitochondrial metabolism, there is an insufficient defense of endogenous antioxidants. In this case, oxidative molecules can disrupt cellular functions by affecting synaptic plasticity, ultimately leading to neuronal injury and apoptosis. Individuals with DS over the age of 35 have a higher frequency of short-term memory impairment and an increase in the rate of dementia, aphasia, and agnosia, while executive function impairments are evident as early as adolescence. One of the most important genes associated with DS is amyloid precursor protein (APP), a gene encoded on chromosome 21. Increased APP production may contribute in part to oxidative stress associated with neurodegenerative diseases and inflammation. Accumulation of amyloid-beta monomers can directly disrupt mitochondrial function resulting in reduced energy and accumulation of amyloid plaques leading to activation of inflammatory cascades [36, 37].

Alzheimer disease (AD) is a form of dementia that can most commonly develop in people with DS, as in the general population. Unfortunately, effective drugs have not yet been developed to be available to treat dementia in DS. Prevention is crucial to alleviate the symptoms of neurodegenerative diseases, but also to delay them. Detection of biomarkers and the development of sensitive cognitive screening tools will be essential for earlier diagnosis and better therapeutic management [38]. There are numerous studies on how to reduce or slow down the course of neurodegenerative diseases, such as AD, in people with DS. The causes of AD in people with DS is associated with overexpression of genes and lack of nutrients due to poor diet can be influenced by regulation of endogenous antioxidants, intake of vitamins, minerals, polyunsaturated fatty acids, and polyphenols [39–42].

5. Commonly used nutritional supplements for individuals with Down syndrome

5.1 Vitamins

As explained in the previous chapter, increased oxidative stress in individuals with DS is present from early life, leading to lipid peroxidation and DNA damage [43]. For that reason, antioxidant vitamins have been the focus of many research (**Table 2**). Vitamin E, especially its form known as α-tocopherol, is a strong antioxidant, important for the prevention of oxidation of unsaturated fatty acids in cell membranes [49, 50]. Some studies involved trisomy 16 mouse models in order to get a basis before clinical trials on DS humans because these mice have increased oxidative stress and cerebral pathology similar to DS [51–54].

Experimental group	Vitamin	Duration of trial	Result	Ref.
Randomized, placebo-controlled study, 20536 adults aged 40–80	600 mg/day vitE 250 mg/day vitamin C 20 mg/day of carotene	5 year treatment period	No improvement in cognitive abilities, no significant differences in all-cause, and vascular and non-vascular mortality.	[44]
93 children with DS aged 7–15 years, 26 non-DS siblings in the same age range as a control group	400 IU vitamin E	4 months	No change in TBARS levels and reduced 8-OHdG levels.	[21]
Randomized double-blind study, 53 individuals with DS	900 IU α-tocoferol, 200 mg ascorbic acid, 600 mg α-lipoic acid	2 years	No improvement or stabilisation of dementia.	[45]
5092 elderly people (90% aged 65 years and older)	Various combinations of vitamin E, C, and multivitamins	3 years	Combination of vitamins gave positive results in prevalence of Alzheimer's disease.	[46]
156 infants aged under 7 months with trisomy 21	100 mg vitamin E, 0 mg vitamin C, 0,9 mg vitamin A, 10 μg Se, 5 mg Zn, and 0,1 mg folinic acid	18 months	No effect on SOD, GPx activity and SOD/GPx ratio, no effect on Griffiths developmental quotient, and an adapted MacArthur communicative development.	[27]
21 children with DS, 18 healthy children	400 mg vitamin E, 500 mg vitamin C	6 months	Decrease of erythrocytic SOD and CAT, and decrease of GPx activity in DS children.	[47]
160 adults with trisomy 21 and 160 healthy, unrelated subjects aged 26 ± 4 years	5 mg/day folic acid, 5 mg/day vitamin B6, 100 μg/day B12 alone or in combination	–	No significant differences in fasting blood tHcy concentrations between healthy controls and adult trisomy 21 patients that justify B vitamin supplementation.	[48]

Table 2.
Examples of vitamin supplementation research for DS individuals.

Lockrow et al. [43] suggested that transgenic mice could be used in order to get insight into the molecular pathways of the disease and to test the efficiency of drugs. They also warned that mice do not manifest all the features as humans do. Still, they proved a correlation between high oxidative stress in transgenic mice and low working memory. The introduction of vitamin E to the diet of mice gave positive results on oxidative stress and neuronal markers. They also suggested that this could be a good starting point for the treatment of neurodegenerative diseases, such as DS and AD, in humans. Lott [55] pointed out that clinical studies on humans still did not provide satisfactory results, although animal studies in oxidative stress are promising.

As presented in **Table 2**, studies on humans had very different experimental groups in the number of participants, age, and dosage of supplements. The conclusions they obtained were also very different. Lockrow et al. [43] and Lott [55] suggested that vitamin E supplementation could exhibit better results if implemented at younger age as preventive therapy for dementia, but it requires additional clinical trials. Tanabe et al. [56] could not find a correlation between elevated Cu-Zn SOD activity and cellular vitamin E status in DS.

It can be seen that a combination of vitamins E and C have been commonly used. Vitamin C helps to maintain a stable concentration of vitamin E in plasma by protecting it from damaging oxidation and keeping it in the active state [49, 57, 58]. The link between cognitive decline in AD and vitamin C intake has been studied by Harrison [18]. He included many studies involving vitamin C or a combination of vitamin C and E in his review article. Contradictory results regarding the usefulness of high doses of vitamin C for the cognitive decline have been provided, but a high connection between the low consummation rate of fruits and vegetables and bad cognitive function has been undoubtfully proved. So, prevention of deficiency by quality nutrition should be the first line of defense against cognitive decline instead of supplementation.

It is very important to remember that high doses of supplements can lead to organ damage, harmful interactions, and toxicity [59]. Besides, reactive oxygen species are necessary for obtaining normal cell functioning, so implementation of high doses of antioxidant supplementation would remove too much ROS disrupting cell signaling pathways [60, 61]. The dietary institute for medicine recommends 22 IU RDA for vitamin E and 75 to 90 mg for vitamin C, which is much lower than the doses usually present in supplements (up to 1000 IU of vitamin E and up to 1000 mg of vitamin C) or which have been used in previously mentioned studies [62].

The deficiency of B12 vitamin is mainly associated with a vegetarian and vegan diet, since it mainly originates from animal products. B12 deficiency in infants can lead to various clinical symptoms, such as hypotonic muscles, involuntary muscle movements, apathy, cerebral atrophy, and demyelination of nerve cells [63, 64]. It has an important role in brain function and development through methylation reactions in the central nervous system. Vitamin B12 is also a cofactor in numerous catalytic reactions in the human body, which are required for neurotransmitter synthesis and functioning. Vitamin B12 deficiency can also result in neuropathy through degeneration of nerve fibers and irreversible brain damage [65]. Folates are also B group, water-soluble vitamins, which serve as coenzymes in a variety of reactions. Numerous enzymes involved in folate transport and metabolism are encoded by genes located on chromosome 21 and represent a potential mechanistic basis for folate dysregulation in children with DS. Potential genetic causes of metabolic folate dysregulation in children with DS, non-genetic factors, such as diet, gender, and age, must be considered because they must fully satisfy their folate needs through their diet since they lack the enzymatic machinery necessary to synthesize their own. There are two possible mechanisms for the influence of folate and vitamin B12 deficiency on the brain: by disrupting myelination or influencing the inflammatory process [66, 67].

Individuals with DS have higher plasma homocysteine concentration than healthy people. There are several possible reasons for changes in its metabolism. The deficiency of vitamin B6, B12, and folic acid is one of the theories explaining the accumulation of homocysteine because those vitamins are important cofactors for its metabolism. High plasma concentration is a result of a high cytotoxic intracellular homocysteine. It is assumed that this is a repercussion of gene overexpression on chromosome 21 [68, 69]. Studies [14, 70–73] proved that intake of high doses of B group vitamins reduced homocysteine levels and reduced the rate of brain atrophy in individuals with mild cognitive deterioration. On the other hand, Fillon-Emery et al. [48] presented results, which showed that the plasma homocysteine concentration of individuals with DS who did not take supplemental vitamins was not significantly different from that of controls. Moretti et al. [74, 75] also warned that research on vitamin B supplementation gives contradictory results without scientific evidence for cognitive improvement.

5.2 ω-3 fatty acids

There are numerous roles of dietary lipids essential for the proper function of cells. They are building material for cellular membranes and bioactive molecules, serve as a source of energy, take part in cell signaling pathways and participate in the regulation of gene expression. Eicosapentaenoic acid (EPA) and docosahexaenoic acid (DHA) are essential polyunsaturated fatty acids with an omega-3 desaturation that cannot be synthesized in the human body [76].

In total, 60% of the dry weight of the human brain are lipids, of which 20% are DHA and arachidonic acid (AA; an omega-6 fatty acid) the two core fatty acids found in gray matter. For that reason, there is a high interest in the influence of unsaturated fatty acids, especially essential ones, for cognitive brain development [77].

Adequate intake of omega-3-fatty acids is crucial for the normal functioning of brain tissue. As already mentioned, as parts of cell membranes, they influence membrane fluidity and modulate ion channels. They are also important in inflammation and immune reactions, as well as for signal processing and neural transmission [77–79].

5.3 Minerals

Due to the fact that SOD and GPx, important enzymes involved in oxidative homeostasis of the cells, contain Se and Zn, these minerals are considered as crucial antioxidant vitamins [80, 81]. Some of the studies about the influence of mentioned minerals on DS individuals are presented in **Table 3**. Besides its role in antioxidative enzymes and metabolism, Se influences serum concentrations of IgG2 and IgG4 in children with DS. DS children are very sensitive to respiratory bacterial infections, and it has been proved that Se concentration decreases after severe bacterial infection. In that light, intake of Se could be beneficial for children with DS as a part of the immune response to bacterial antigens [89]. Se is also important for the production of thyroid hormones. The thyroid gland tissue contains a high concentration of Se [90]. In the case of Se deficiency, H_2O_2 gets accumulated and oxidative stress increases that lead to cell apoptosis [91]. Adequate Se intake is necessary for proper intracellular GPx functioning and protection of thyrocytes from peroxides [26]. Hypothyroidism is common in people with DS, so Se supplementation could be useful in that case [92]. The same as already mentioned for vitamins, adequate intake of Se by proper diet should be considered first. The bioavailability of Se originating from proteinaceous food (meat, fish, shellfish, eggs, and cereals) varies from 20% to 80% (the best is from cereals and yeast). It is mainly in the form of selenomethionine. In supplements, the inorganic form of Se, sodium selenite, is mainly used and has excellent bioavailability [91, 93, 94].

Zinc deficiency slows growth because it is involved in the activity of more than 200 enzymes, especially those associated with the synthesis of RNA and DNA. It is important for the function of numerous enzymes and transcription factors [95].

Experimental and clinical studies have found that zinc metabolism is altered in individuals with Down syndrome (**Table 3**). Lima et al. [85], reported that adequate

Experimental group	Mineral	Duration of trial	Result	Ref.
29 trisomy 21 patients 9 to 36 years and 32 age-matched controls	Measurement of Zn, Cu, and Se level	–	Mean plasma Zn and Cu level of DS subjects were not different from that of the control group. Mean plasma Se was significantly decreased in DS subjects, and activity of GPx was significantly increased in the DS group.	[82]
Group aged 1 to 54 years	Supplementation of Na–selenite in a dose of 0.015–0.025 mg/kg/day	0.3–1.5 years	GPx activity increased by 25%, and the SOD1/GPx ratio decreased by 23.9% in the Se group.	[83]
18 DS children aged from 8 months to 3 years with trisomy 21, translocations, and mosaicism, and control group of 15 children	Measurement of the activities of SOD and GPx, and the levels of their cofactors Cu, Zn, and Se	–	Insufficient concentrations of Se in individuals with DS, Cu levels significantly higher in DS groups, and plasma Zn concentrations were normal. Whole-blood Se levels were decreased significantly in all patients compared to controls, with no correlation between whole Se levels and GPx activity. SOD and GPx activity do not show a correlation with clinical manifestations of DS.	[84]
35 children with DS and 33 controls both aged 4–11 years	Zn in plasma, urine, and erythrocyte	–	Decreased Zn levels in the plasma and urine of DS subjects in comparison to the control group, and erythrocyte Zn levels were adequate.	[85]
30 children with Down syndrome	Measurement of Zn level	5 years	Up to 5 years of age, plasma Zn levels are adequate but tend to decrease after this age.	[86]
38 DS children 2–15 years old, 20 healthy children aged 2–14 years	Measurement of serum concentration of Zn and Ig before and after 20 mg/kg/day of zinc sulfate for two months.	2 years	Low plasma Zn levels in DS patients, but no correlation was found between the Zn deficiency and the recurrence or intensity of infections. Low serum Zn levels in some DS children increased after supplementation. No difference between DS children and control in the percentage of B lymphocytes, and serum IgG, IgA, and IgM levels.	[87]
19 children with DS 2–6 years old and 11 age-matched controls	Measurement of hair zinc levels	–	Hair zinc levels are significantly lower in those with Down syndrome.	[88]

Table 3.
Examples of research on mineral status in DS individuals.

zinc intake was observed in 40% of children with DS and in 67% of the control group and zinc concentrations were significantly lower in plasma and urine and higher in erythrocytes of children with DS. There are several possible reasons for that: low plasma Zn concentration could be a result of a redistribution of a mineral in an organism, and not an inhibition of its absorption. A high level of erythrocytes Zn may be a consequence of increased Cu-Zn SOD activity. If DS children are iron deficient (which occurs quite often), Zn binds to the protoporphyrin instead of the iron [85]. Many symptoms of children and adults with DS are a consequence of excessive synthesis of multiple gene products, including an increase in the intracellular activity of Cu-Zn SOD due to overexpression of genes present on chromosome 21. Zinc stabilizes the 3D structure of SOD, and, thus reduces the imbalance [85]. It also participates in the formation of thyroid hormones, leucocytes, and antibodies [49, 96, 97].

5.4 Polyphenols

Mitochondria are the primary site for the creation of free radicals due to the production of adenosine triphosphate (ATP) through oxidative phosphorylation (OXPHOS), so elevated oxidative stress in individuals with DS primarily affects these organelles. DS individuals have decreased efficiency in producing ATP and reduced respiratory capacity. Mitochondria dysfunction primarily influence brain functioning because of its high susceptibility to energy deficit [98].

Epigallocatechin gallate (EGCG) originating from green tea has been studied in mouse and cell models, and it has been found that it is effective as a ROS scavenging agent, mitochondrial apoptosis protector, mitochondrial bioenergetics activator, and respiratory chain promotor [98, 99]. On the other hand, *in vivo* tests found that EGCG bioavailability is low, due to poor absorption and metabolic modification. It is still unknown whether metabolites reach the brain and influence cell metabolism [99]. Torre and Dierssen [75] warned that many clinical trials in DS patients have limitations, such as poor design, a reduced number of participants, a lack of methods for the neuropsychological evaluation of patients, and the dependence on the IQ of individuals.

It is considered that concentrations of polyphenols normally present in foods are too low to exhibit a beneficial effect on metabolic pathways, so supplementation should be implemented in the daily routine of individuals with DS [100]. This opens an important question about the dosage. Namely, EGCG in high doses acts as a prooxidant with harmful effects on skeletal DS phenotypes, liver, kidney, thymus, spleen, and pancreas [101, 102]. 10 mg/kg/day of EGCG has been found as safe, and effective on mitochondrial and behavioral dysfunction by a case study on a 10-year-old DS child. Although studies on mouse models targeted doses of 10/mg/kg/day–50 mg/kg/day as harmful without positive effect [100]. Long et al. [102] in his survey found that commercially available preparations ranged from 351 mg/day to 2000 mg/day. Some respondents included in this survey reported improvement in speech, memory, learning, and energy, while the others quit supplementation due to the lack of improvements.

Research provided by Xicota et al. [103] tried to determine the influence of EGCG supplementation (9 mg/kg) on body weight. It is considered that EGCG decreases the absorption of lipids and glucose. The survey followed the DS group during 12 months of supplementation and additional 6 months after quitting the treatment. Male subjects exhibited less body weight gain, unlike female subjects, but the authors did not provide an explanation for such results and further research should be done in order to confirm these findings.

Resveratrol originating from different berries, grapes, red wine, and peanuts is another polyphenol used as a therapy for the improvement of mitochondrial functions and diminishing some of the DS clinical features [100]. The same as already mentioned for EGCG, bioavailability is low and its original form quickly changes into metabolites [104]. Studies on the experimental rats determined doses of 700 mg/kg/day as safe [104]. Considering the fact that it is not the resveratrol that reaches targeted tissues but its metabolites, those molecules should be the focus of research in future as a treatment for DS.

5.5 Choline and CoQ10 supplementation

Choline is an essential nutrient that has to be derived from the diet. Although it can be synthesized in the body, this is not sufficient to support bodily needs [105, 106]. Choline supply is critical for brain development because it is a precursor of acetylcholine—a key neurotransmitter for regulating neuronal proliferation, maturation, plasticity, survival, and synapse formation. Besides this, choline is the precursor of phosphatidylcholine and sphingomyelin—principal components of neuronal and other cellular membranes. It is also a primary dietary source of methyl groups in humans [107]. It acts as a methyl donor through the betaine–methionine pathway. Alterations in the dietary levels of choline during early development can produce life-long effects on gene expression through DNA methylation [108].

Disturbances in the cholinergic system are likely due to alterations in acetylcholine metabolism with a significant relationship to AD-like symptoms in DS adults since an impaired acetylcholine metabolism has been reported in the brains of individuals with AD. A reduction in the cholinergic neurotransmitter choline acetyltransferase has also been reported in cortical and sub-cortical regions of DS adult brain tissues [53]. Cholinergic deficits in the brain are a hallmark in humans with DS and Ts16 mice. Brains of DS individuals exhibit a significant reduction in choline acetyltransferase activity in the cerebral cortex, which is consistent with the impaired development of the basal forebrain cholinergic system exhibited by Ts16 mice [109].

So far, there is no evidence that choline supplementation possibly improves cognitive functioning when given to young or adult individuals with DS [110]. On the other hand, several studies proved that perinatal choline supplementation in Ts65Dn mice has beneficial effects on Ts65Dn offspring, including improvements in attention, emotion regulation, spatial memory, and the protection of cholinergic neurons in the medial septal nucleus (MSN) [107, 108, 111]. Specific molecular mechanisms by which supplementing the maternal diet with additional choline exerts life-long effects on offspring functioning are not clear yet, and further studies are necessary [112]. It is believed that it enhances the target-derived neuroprotection of Ts65Dn basal forebrain cholinergic neurons (BFCNs), which typically begin to atrophy at six months of age due to the impaired retrograde transport of nerve growth factor (NGF) [108]. Although Ts65Dn mice do not show all the genetic and phenotypic features of DS, these findings suggest the interesting possibility that increased maternal choline intake during pregnancy may represent a safe and beneficial intervention at the earliest stages [107]. Nevertheless, results obtained in mice tests suggest that current dietary guidelines for choline (425 mg/day for women and450 mg/day for pregnant women) [106], which are necessary to prevent liver damage, may not be sufficient for brain development and higher levels should be taken during pregnancy [110].

Coenzyme Q10 (CoQ10) is lyophilic quinone that can be synthesized by an organism or introduced by the diet. His cell functions include antioxidant activity, carrying

Experimental group	Dosage of CoQ10	Duration of trial	Result	Ref.
30 DS patients	4 mg/kg/day	6 months	CoQ10 treatment was not able to revert DNA damage in heavily compromised cells, while being able to minimize DNA damage in lightly damaged cells.	[114]
17 DS patients 5 to 17 years old	4 mg/kg/day	20 months	Treatment resulted in a significant rise of Co10 in plasma, but it did not affect the overall extent of DNA damage.	[115]
32 DS patients	CoQ10 in a form of ubiquinone (reduced form) in a concentration 4 mg/kg/day	4 years	Long-term treatment did not affect DNA or RNA oxidation in children with DS.	[116]

Table 4.
Examples of CoQ10 supplementation research for DS individuals.

electrons in mitochondria, and serving as a cofactor to some enzymes [113]. There is a theory that CoQ10 could diminish oxidative DNA damage and serve as a therapy for issues related to DS. Research examples presented in **Table 4** show that an additional survey should be conducted in order to confirm this theory.

6. Conclusions

Education and encouragement of caregivers of people with DS to pay attention to the quality of nutrition should be the focus of professionals included in DS rehabilitation. Prevention of nutrient deficiency is certainly cheaper and more effective than dealing with supplementation. Since the metabolic pathways of people with DS are altered, they are more sensitive to nutrient deficiencies than the rest of the population. So, nutrient status should be a part of routine health screening and supplementation should be introduced only after deficiencies of certain nutrients have been identified. Supplementation should be introduced only as directed by a physician. Many research has shown promising results about the improvement of health status and intellectual development of individuals with DS, but the safety of doses and their efficiency have not been proved by independent scientific studies, especially in relation to the diet and nutrient status of DS individuals prior to supplementation.

Conflict of interest

The authors declare no conflict of interest.

Author details

Maja Ergović Ravančić and Valentina Obradović*
Polytechic in Požega, Vukovarska, Pozega, Croatia

*Address all correspondence to: vobradovic@vup.hr

References

[1] Glaw S, Platt L. Trisomy 21. In: Copel J, D'Alton M, Feltovich H, et al., editors. Obstetic Imaging: Fetal Diagnosis and Care. 2nd ed. Philadelphia, USA: Elsevier; 2018. pp. 608-613. DOI: 10.1016/C2014-0-00100-1

[2] Park J, Chung KC. New perspectives of Dyrk1A role in neurogenesis and neuropathologic features of Down syndrome. Experimental Neurobiology. 2013;**22**:244-248. DOI: 10.5607/en.2013.22.4.244

[3] Salman M. Systematic review of the effect of therapeutic dietary supplements and drugs on cognitive function in subjects with Down syndrome. European Journal of Paediatric Neurology. 2002;**6**:213-219. DOI: 10.1053/ejpn.2002.0596

[4] Malini SS. Ramachandra: NB Influence of advanced age of maternal grandmothers on Down Syndrome. BMC Medical Genetics. 2006;**7**:4-8

[5] Diamandopoulos K, Green J. Down syndrome: An integrative review. Journal of Neonatal Nursing. 2018;**24**:235-241. DOI: 10.1016/j.jnn.2018.01.001

[6] Bertapelli F, Pitetti K, Agiovlasitis S, Guerra-Junior G. Overweight and obesity in children and adolescents with Down syndrome—prevalence, determinants, consequences, and interventions: A literature review. Research in Developmental Disabilities. 2016;**57**:181-192. DOI: 10.1016/j.ridd.2016.06.018

[7] Haydar TF, Reeves RH. Trisomy 21 and early brain development. Trends in Neurosciences. 2012;**35**:81-91. DOI: 10.1016/j.tins.2011.11.001

[8] Asim A, Kumar A, Muthuswamy S, Jain S, Agarwal S. Down syndrome: An insight of the disease. Journal of Biomedical Science. 2015;**22**(1):41. DOI: 10.1186/s12929-015-0138-y

[9] Eckdahl TT. Down Syndrome: One Smart Cookie. New York, USA: Momentum Press; 2018

[10] Roccatello G, Cocchi G, Dimastromatteo RT, Cavallo A, Biserni GB, Selicati M, et al. Eating and lifestyle habits in youth with Down syndrome attending a care program: An exploratory lesson for future improvements. Frontiers in Nutrition. 2021;**8**:641112. DOI: 10.3389/fnut.2021.641112

[11] Cooley C. Nonconventional therapies for Down syndrome: A review and framework for decision making. In: Cohen W, Nadel L, Madnick M, editors. Down Syndrome Visions for the 21st century. 1st ed. New York, USA: Wiley-Liss, Inc; 2002. pp. 608-613

[12] Sacks B, Buckley F. Multi-nutrient formulas and other substances as therapies for Down syndrome: An overview. Down Syndrome News and Update. 1998;**1**:70-83

[13] Fish Q. The history of targeted nutritional intervention. In: Fish K, Fish Q, editors. Down Syndrome: What You Can Do. USA: Qadoshyah Fish. Moodys; 2008. pp. 87-89

[14] Ani C, Grantham-McGregor S, Muller D. Nutritional supplementation in Down syndrome: Theoretical considerations and current status. Developmental Medicine and Child Neurology. 2000;**42**:207-213. DOI: 10.1017/s0012162200000359

[15] Roizen NJ. Complementary and alternative therapies for Down

syndrome. Mental Retardation and Developmental Disabilities Research Reviews. 2005;**11**:149-155. DOI: 10.1002/mrdd.20063

[16] Lewanda AF, Gallegos MF, Summar M. Patterns of dietary supplement use in children with Down syndrome. The Journal of Pediatrics. 2018;**201**:100-105. DOI: 10.1016/j.jpeds.2018.05.022

[17] Guilford F, Hope J. Deficient glutathione in the pathophysiology of mycotoxin-related illness. Toxins. 2014;**6**:608-623. DOI: 10.3390/toxins6020608

[18] Harrison FE. A critical review of vitamin C for the prevention of age-related cognitive decline and Alzheimer's disease. Journal of Azheimers Disease. 2012;**29**:711-726. DOI: 10.3233/JAD-2012-111853

[19] Barone E, Arena A, Head E, Butterfield DA, Perluigi M. Disturbance of redox homeostasis in Down Syndrome: Role of iron dysmetabolism. Free Radical Biology & Medicine. 2018;**114**:84-93. DOI: 10.1016/j.freeradbiomed.2017.07.009

[20] Komatsu T, Duckyoung Y, Ito A, Kurosawa K, Maehata Y, Kubodera T, et al. Increased oxidative stress biomarkers in the saliva of Down syndrome patients. Archives of Oral Biology. 2013;**58**:1246-1250. DOI: 10.1016/j.archoralbio.2013.03.017

[21] Nachvak SM, Neyestani TR, Mahboob SA, Sabour S, Keshawarz SA. Speakman JR: α-Tocopherol supplementation reduces biomarkers of oxidative stress in children with Down syndrome: A randomized controlled trial. European Journal of Clinical Nutrition. 2014;**68**:1119-1123. DOI: 10.1038/ejcn.2014.97

[22] Garlet TR, Parisotto EB, de Medeiros S, Pereira LC, Moreira EA, Dalmarco EM, et al. Systemic oxidative stress in children and teenagers with Down syndrome. Life Sciences. 2013;**93**:558-563. DOI: 10.1016/j.lfs.2013.08.017

[23] Ferreira M, Rodrigues R, Motta E, Debom G, Soares F, de Mattos BS, et al. Evaluation of extracellular adenine nucleotides hydrolysis in platelets and biomarkers of oxidative stress in Down syndrome individuals. Biomedicine & Pharmacotherapy. 2015;**74**:200-205. DOI: 10.1016/j.biopha.2015.08.007

[24] Liochev SI, Fridovich I. Mechanism of the peroxidase activity of Cu, Zn superoxide dismutase. Free Radical Biology & Medicine. 2010;**48**:1565-1569. DOI: 10.1016/j.freeradbiomed.2010.02.036

[25] Shields N, Downs J, de Haan JB, Taylor NF, Torr J, Fernhall B, et al. What effect does regular exercise have on oxidative stress in people with Down syndrome? A systematic review with meta-analyses. Journal of Science and Medicine in Sport. 2018;**21**:596-603

[26] Campos C, Casado Á. Oxidative stress, thyroid dysfunction & Down syndrome. Indian Journal of Medical Research. 2015;**142**:113-119

[27] Ellis JM, Tan HK, Gilbert RE, Muller DPR, Henley W, Moy R, et al. Supplementation with antioxidants and folinic acid for children with Down's syndrome: Randomised controlled trial. British Medical Journal. 2008;**336**:594-597. DOI: 10.1136/bmj.39465.544028.AE

[28] Pinto M, Neves J, Palha M, Bicho M. Oxidative stress in Portuguese children with Down syndrome. Down's Syndrome, Research and Practice. 2002;**8**:79-82. DOI: 10.3104/reports.134

[29] Sulthana SM, Kumar SN, Sridhar MG, Bhat BV, Rao KR. Levels of nonenzymatic antioxidants in Down syndrome. The Indian Journal of Pediatrics. 2012;**79**:1473-1476. DOI: 10.1007/s12098-012-0795-8

[30] Strydom A, Dickinson MJ, Shende S, Pratico D, Walker Z. Oxidative stress and cognitive ability in adults with Down syndrome. Progress in Neuro-Psychopharmacology & Biological Psychiatry. 2009;**33**:76-80. DOI: 10.1016/j.pnpbp.2008.10.006

[31] Nagy Z, Westerberg H, Klingberg T. Maturation of white matter is associated with the development of cognitive functions during childhood. Journal of Cognitive Neuroscience. 2004;**16**: 1227-1233. DOI: 10.1162/ 0898929041920441

[32] Giedd J, Stockman M, Weddle C, Liverpool M, Alexander-Bloch A, Wallace G, et al. Anatomic magnetic resonance imaging of the developing child and adolescent brain and effects of genetic variation. Neuropsychology Review. 2010;**20**:349-361. DOI: 10.1007/ s11065-010-9151-9

[33] Bryan J, Osendarp S, Hughes D, Calvaresi E, Baghurst K, Van Klinken JW. Nutrients for cognitive development in school-aged children. Nutrition Reviews. 2004;**62**:295-306. DOI: 10.1111/j.1753-4887.2004.tb00055.x

[34] Benton D. Overview of an emerging field. In: Prasad C, Lieberman H, Kanarek R, editors. Nutrition, Brain & Behavior. Boca Raton: Taylor and Francis; 2005. pp. 57-71

[35] Benton D. The Influence of dietary status on the cognitive performance of children. Molecular Nutrition & Food Research. 2010;**54**:457-470. DOI: 10.1002/mnfr.200900158

[36] Lockrow JP, Ashley M, Fortress AM, Granholm AE. Age-related neurodegeneration and memory loss in Down syndrome. Current Gerontology and Geriatrics Research. 2012;**2012**:463909. DOI: 10.1155/2012/463909

[37] Lott IT, Head E. Alzheimer disease and Down syndrome: Factors in pathogenesis. Neurobiology of Aging. 2005;**26**:383-389. DOI: 10.1016/j. neurobiolaging.2004.08.005

[38] Caraci F, Iulita MF, Pentz R, Aguilar LF, Orciani C, Barone C, et al. Searching for new pharmacological targets for the treatment of Alzheimer's disease in Down syndrome. European Journal of Pharmacology. 2017;**15**:7-19. DOI: 10.1016/j.ejphar.2017.10.004

[39] Zana M, Janka Z. Oxidative stress: A bridge between Down Syndrome and Alzheimer's disease. Neurobiology of Aging. 2007;**28**:648-676

[40] Laurin D, Masaki KH, Foley DJ, White LR, Launer LJ. Midlife dietary intake of antioxidants and risk of late-life incident dementia: The Honolulu-Asia Aging Study. American Journal of Epidemiology. 2004;**159**:959-967. DOI: 10.1093/aje/kwh124

[41] Clarke R, Harrison G, Richards S. Effect of vitamins and aspirin on markers of platelet activation, oxidative stress and homocysteine in people at high risk of dementia. Journal of Internal Medicine. 2003;**254**:67-75. DOI: 10.1046/j.1365-2796.2003.01154.x

[42] Planas M, Conde M, Audivert S, Perez-Portabella C, Burgos R, Chacon P, et al. Micronutrient supplementation in mild Alzheimer disease patients. Clinical Nutrition. 2004;**23**:265-272

[43] Lockrow J, Prakasam A, Huang P, Bimonte-Nelson H, Sambamurti K,

Granholm AC. Cholinergic degeneration and memory loss delayed by vitamin E in a Down syndrome mouse model. Experimental Neurology. 2009;**216**(2):278-289. DOI: 10.1016/j.expneurol.2008.11.021

[44] Heart Protection Study Collaborative Group. MRC/BHF Heart Protection Study of antioxidant vitamin supplementation in 20,536 high-risk individuals: A randomised placebo-controlled trial. The Lancet. 2002;**360**:23-33. DOI: 10.1016/S0140-6736(02)09328-5

[45] Lott IT, Doran E, Nguyen VQ, Tournay A, Head E, Gillen DL. Down syndrome and dementia: A randomized, controlled trial of antioxidant supplementation. American Journal of Medical Genetics Part. 2011;**155A**:1939-1948. DOI: 10.1002/ajmg.a.34114

[46] Zandi PP, Anthony JC, Khachaturian AS, Stone SV, Gustafson D, Tschanz JT, et al. Reduced risk of Alzheimer disease in users of antioxidant vitamin supplements: The Cache County Study. Archives of Neurology. 2004;**61**:82-88. DOI: 10.1001/archneur.61.1.82

[47] Parisotto EB, Garlet TR, Cavalli VL, Zamoner A, da Rosa JS, Bastos J, et al. Antioxidant intervention attenuates oxidative stress in children and teenagers with Down syndrome. Research in Developmental Disabilities. 2014;**35**:1228-1236. DOI: 10.1016/j.ridd.2014.03.013

[48] Fillon-Emery N, Chango A, Mircher C, Barbé F, Bléhaut H, Herbeth B, et al. Homocysteine concentrations in adults with trisomy 21: Effect of B vitamins and genetic polymorphisms. The American Journal of Clinical Nutrition. 2004;**80**:1551-1557. DOI: 10.1093/ajcn/80.6.1551

[49] Arsic B, Dimitrijevic D, Kostic D. Mineral and vitamin fortification. In: Grumezescu AM, editor. Nutraceuticals Nanotechnology in the Agri-food Industry. 1st ed. San Diego, USA: Elsevier; 2016. pp. 1-40

[50] Brigelius-Flohe R. Bioactivity of vitamin E. Nutrition Research Reviews. 2006;**19**:174-186. DOI: 10.1017/S0954422407202938

[51] Bartesaghi R, Guidi S, Ciani E. Is it possible to improve neurodevelopmental abnormalities in Down syndrome? Reviews in the Neurosciences. 2011;**22**:419-455. DOI: 10.1515/RNS.2011.037

[52] Mowery CT, Reyes JM, et al. Trisomy of a Down syndrome critical region globally amplifies transcription via HMGN1 overexpression. Cell Reports. 2018;**25**:1898-1911. DOI: 10.1016/j.celrep.2018.10.061

[53] Vacca RA, Bawari S, Valenti D, Tewari D, Nabavi SF, Shirooie S, et al. Down syndrome: Neurobiological alterations and therapeutic targets. Neuroscience and Biobehavioral Reviews. 2019;**98**:234-255. DOI: 10.1016/j.neubiorev.2019.01.001

[54] Bambrick LL, Fiskum G. Mitochondrial dysfunction in mouse trisomy 16 brain. Brain Research. 2008;**1188**:9-16. DOI: 10.1016/j.brainres.2007.10.045

[55] Lott IT. Antioxidants in Down syndrome. Biochimica et Biophysica Acta. 2012;**1822**:657-663. DOI: 10.1016/j.bbadis.2011.12.010

[56] Tanabe T, Kawamura N, Morinobu T, Murata T, Tamai H, Mino M, et al. Antioxidant enzymes and vitamins in Down's syndrome. Pathophysiology. 1994;**1**:93-97. DOI: 10.1016/0928-4680(94)90022-1

[57] Rizvi S, Raza ST, Ahmed F, Abbas S, Mahdi F. The role of Vitamin E in human health and some diseases. Sultan Qaboos University Medical Journal. 2014;**14**:157-165

[58] Wintergerst ES, Maggini S, Hornig DH. Immune-enhancing role of Vitamin C and zinc and effect on clinical conditions. Annals of Nutrition & Metabolism. 2006;**50**:85-94. DOI: 10.1159/000090495

[59] Binns CW, Lee MK, Lee AH. Problems and prospects: Public health regulation of dietary supplements. Annual Review of Public Health. 2018;**39**:403-420. DOI: 10.1146/annurev-publhealth-040617-013638

[60] Kurutas EB. The importance of antioxidants which play the role in cellular response against oxidative/nitrosative stress: Current state. Nutrition Journal. 2016;**15**:71-93. DOI: 10.1186/s12937-016-0186-5

[61] Landete JM. Dietary intake of natural antioxidants: Vitamins and polyphenols. Critical Reviews in Food Science and Nutrition. 2013;**53**:706-721. DOI: 10.1080/10408398.2011.555018

[62] Ergović Ravančić M, Obradović V. Usage of nutritional supplements for individuals with Down syndrome. Progress in Nutrition. 2021;**23**:1-20

[63] Louwman MW, van Dusseldorp M, van de Vijver FJ, Thomas CM, Schneede J, Ueland PM, et al. Signs of impaired cognitive function in adolescents with marginal cobalamin status. The American Journal of Clinical Nutrition. 2000;**72**:762-769. DOI: 10.1093/ajcn/72.3.762

[64] Nyaradi A, Li J, Hickling S, Foster J, Oddy WH. The role of nutrition in children's neurocognitive development, from pregnancy through childhood. Frontiers in Human Neuroscience. 2013;7:1-16. DOI: 10.3389/fnhum.2013.00097

[65] Winje BA, Kvestad I, Krishnamachari S, Manji K, Taneja S, Bellinger DC, et al. Does early vitamin B12 supplementation improve neurodevelopment and cognitive function in childhood and into school age: A study protocol for extended follow-ups from randomised controlled trials in India and Tanzania. BMJ Open. 2018;**8**:1-9. DOI: 10.1136/bmjopen-2017-018962

[66] Pfeiffer CM, Hughes JP, Lacher DA, Bailey RL, Berry RJ, Zhang M, et al. Estimation of trends in serum and RBC folate in the U.S. population from pre- to postfortification using assay-adjusted data from the NHANES 1988-2010. Journal of Nutrition. 2012;**142**:886-893

[67] Black MM. Effects of vitamin B12 and folate deficiency on brain development in children. Food and Nutrition Bulletin. 2008;**29**:126-131. DOI: 10.1177/15648265080292S117

[68] Engelborghs S, Gilles C, Ivanoiu A, Vandewoude M. Rationale and clinical data supporting nutritional intervention in Alzheimer's disease. Acta Clinica Belgica. 2014;**69**:17-24. DOI: 10.1179/0001551213Z.0000000006

[69] Pogribna M, Melnyk S, Pogribny I, Chango A, Yi P, James SJ. Homocysteine metabolism in children with Down syndrome: In vitro modulation. The American Journal of Human Genetics. 2001;**69**:88-95. DOI: 10.1086/321262

[70] Pietruszka B, Brzozowska A. Folic acid supplementation practice in Europe – plenary lectur. Polish Journal of Food and Nutrition Sciences. 2006;**15**:93-99

[71] Smith AD. The worldwide challenge of the dementias: A role for B vitamins and homocysteine? Food and Nutrition Bulletin. 2008;**29**:143-172. DOI: 10.1177/15648265080292S119

[72] Smith AD, Refsum H. Homocysteine, B vitamins, and cognitive impairment. Annual Review of Nutrition. 2016;**36**:211-239. DOI: 10.1146/annurev-nutr-071715-050947

[73] Tinelli C, Di Pino A, Ficulle E, Marcelli S, Feligioni M. Hyperhomocysteinemia as a risk factor and potential nutraceutical target for certain pathologies. Frontiers in Nutrition. 2019;**6**:1-13. DOI: 10.3389/fnut.2019.00049

[74] Moretti R, Caruso P. The controversial role of homocysteine in neurology: From labs to clinical practice. International Journal of Molecular Sciences. 2019;**20**:1-22. DOI: 10.3390/ijms20010231

[75] de la Torre R, Dierssen M. Therapeutic approaches in the improvement of cognitive performance in Down syndrome: Past, present, and future. Progress in Brain Research. 2012;**197**:1-14. DOI: 10.1016/B978-0-444-54299-1.00001-7

[76] Youdim KA, Martin A, Joseph JA. Essential fatty acids and the brain: Possible health implications. International Journal of Developmental Neuroscience. 2000;**18**:383-399. DOI: 10.1016/s0736-5748(00)00013-7

[77] De Souza AS, Fernandes FS, Do Carmo MG. Effects of maternal malnutrition and postnatal nutritional rehabilitation on brain fatty acids, learning, and memory. Nutrition Reviews. 2011;**69**:132-144. DOI: 10.1111/j.1753-4887.2011.00374.x

[78] Schuchardt J, Huss M, Stauss-Grabo M, Hahn A. Significance of long-chain polyunsaturated fatty acids (PUFAs) for the development and behaviour of children. European Journal of Pediatrics. 2010;**169**:149-164. DOI: 10.1007/s00431-009-1035-8

[79] Prado EL, Dewey KG. Nutrition and brain development in early life. Nutrition Reviews. 2014;**72**:267-284. DOI: 10.1111/nure.12102

[80] Holben DH, Smith AM. The diverse role of selenium within selenoproteins: A review. Journal of the American Dietetic Association. 1999;**99**:836-843. DOI: 10.1016/S0002-8223(99)00198-4

[81] Huang Z, Rose AH, Hoffmann PR. The role of selenium in inflammation and immunity: From molecular mechanisms to therapeutic opportunities. Antioxidants & Redox Signaling. 2012;**16**:705-743. DOI: 10.1089/ars.2011.4145

[82] Nève J, Sinet PM, Molle L, Nicole A. Selenium, zinc and copper in Down's syndrome (trisomy 21): Blood levels and relations with glutathione peroxidase and superoxide dismutase. Clinica Chimica Acta. 1983;**133**:209-214. DOI: 10.1016/0009-8981(83)90406-0

[83] Antila E, Nordberg UR, Syväoja EL, Westermarck T. Selenium therapy in Down syndrome (DS): A theory and a clinical trial. Advanced in Experimental Medical Biology. 1990;**264**:183-186. DOI: 10.1007/978-1-4684-5730-8_29

[84] Meguid NA, Kholoussi NM, Afifi HH. Evaluation of superoxide dismutase and glutathione peroxidase enzymes and their cofactors in Egyptian children with Down's syndrome. Biological Trace Element Research. 2001;**81**:21-28. DOI: 10.1385/BTER:81:1:21

[85] Lima AS, Cardoso BR, Cozzolino SF. Nutritional status of zinc in children

with Down syndrome. Biological Trace Element Research. 2010;**133**:20-28. DOI: 10.1007/s12011-009-8408-8

[86] Cocchi G, Mastrocola M, Capelli M, Bastelli A, Vitali F, Corvaglia L. Immunological patterns in young children with Down syndrome: Is there a temporal trend? Acta Paediatrica. 2007;**96**(10):1479-1482. DOI: 10.1111/j.1651-2227.2007.00459.x

[87] Stabile A, Pesaresi MA, Stabile AM, Pastore M, Sopo SM, Ricci R, et al. Immunodeficiency and plasma zinc levels in children with Down's syndrome: A long-term follow-up of oral zinc supplementation. Clinical Immunology and Immunopathology. 1991;**58**(2):207-216. DOI: 10.1016/0090-1229(91)90137-Y

[88] Yenigun A, Ozkinay F, Cogulu O, Coker C, Cetiner N, Ozden G, et al. Hair zinc level in Down syndrome. Down's Syndrome, Research and Practice. 2004;**9**:53-57. DOI: 10.3104/reports.292

[89] Anneren G, Magnusson CGM, Nordvall SL. Increase in serum concentrations of IgG2 and IgG4 by selenium supplementation in children with Down's syndrome. Archives of Disease in Childhood. 1990;**65**:1353-1355. DOI: 10.1136/adc.65.12.1353

[90] Ventura M, Melo M, Carrilho F. Selenium and thyroid disease: From pathophysiology to treatment. International Journal of Endocrinology. 2017;**2017**:1-9. DOI: 10.1155/2017/1297658

[91] Drutel A, Archambeaud F, Caron P. Selenium and the thyroid gland: More good news for clinicians. Clinical Endocrinology. 2013;**78**:155-164. DOI: 10.1111/cen.12066

[92] Thiel R, Fowkes SW. Down syndrome and thyroid dysfunction: Should nutritional support be the first-line treatment? Medical Hypotheses. 2007;**69**:809-815. DOI: 10.1016/j.mehy.2007.01.068

[93] Bhagvan NV, Ha CE. Essentials of Medical Biochemistry. 2nd ed. San Diego, USA: Elsevier; 2015

[94] Caraci F, Iulita MF, Pentz R, Flores Aguilar L, Orciani C, Barone C, et al. Searching for new pharmacological targets for the treatment of Alzheimer's disease in Down syndrome. European Journal of Pharmacology. 2017;**817**:7-19. DOI: 10.1016/j.ejphar.2017.10.004

[95] Mocchegiani E, Bertoni-Freddari C, Marcellini F, Malavolta M. Brain, aging and neurodegeneration: Role of zinc ion availability. Progress in Neurobiology. 2005;**75**:367-390. DOI: 10.1016/j.pneurobio.2005.04.005

[96] Prasad AS. Zinc: Role in immunity, oxidative stress and chronic inflammation. Current Opinion in Clinical Nutrition and Metabolic Care. 2009;**12**:646-652. DOI: 10.1097/MCO.0b013e3283312956

[97] Haase H, Overbeck S, Rink L. Zinc supplementation for the treatment or prevention of disease: Current status and future perspectives. Experimental Gerontology. 2008;**43**:394-408. DOI: 10.1016/j.exger.2007.12.002

[98] Valenti D, Braidy N, De Rasmo D, Signorile A, Rossi L, Georgiev Atanasov A, et al. Mitochondria as pharmacological targets in Down syndrome. Free Radical Biology & Medicine. 2018;**114**:69-83. DOI: 10.1016/j.freeradbiomed.2017.08.014

[99] Vacca RA, Valenti D, Caccamese S, Daglia M, Braidy N, Nabavi SM. Plant polyphenols as natural drugs for the management of Down syndrome and related disorders. Neuroscience and

Biobehavioral Reviews. 2016;**71**:865-877. DOI: 10.1016/j.neubiorev.2016.10.023

[100] Valenti D, de Bari L, de Rasmo D, Signorile A, Henrion-Caude A, Contestabile A, et al. The polyphenols resveratrol and epigallocatechin-3-gallate restore the severe impairment of mitochondria in hippocampal progenitor cells from a Down syndrome mouse model. Biochimica et Biophysica Acta. 1862;**2016**:1093-1104. DOI: 10.1016/j.bbadis.2016.03.003

[101] Vacca RA, Valenti D. Green tea EGCG plus fish oil omega-3 dietary supplements rescue mitochondrial dysfunctions and are safe in a Down's syndrome child. Clinical Nutrition. 2015;**34**:783-784. DOI: 10.1016/j.clnu.2015.04.012

[102] Long R, Drawbaugh ML, Davis CM, Goodlett CR, Williams JR, Roper RJ. Usage of and attitudes about green tea extract and Epigallocathechin-3-gallate (EGCG) as a therapy in individuals with Down syndrome. Complementary Therapies in Medicine. 2019;**45**:234-241. DOI: 10.1016/j.ctim.2019.07.002

[103] Xicota L, Rodríguez J, Langohr K, Fitó M, Dierssen M, de la Torre R. Effect of epigallocatechin gallate on the body composition and lipid profile of Down syndrome individuals: Implications for clinical management. Clinical Nutrition. 2020;**39**:1292-1300. DOI: 10.1016/j.clnu.2019.05.028

[104] Fernandez-Mar MI, Mateos R, Garcia-Parrilla MC, Puertas B, Cantos-Villar E. Bioactive compounds in wine: Resveratrol, hydroxytyrosol and melatonin: A review. Food Chemistry. 2012;**130**:797-813. DOI: 10.1016/j.foodchem.2011.08.023

[105] Lakshmi KT, Surekha RH, Srikanth B, Jyothy A. Serum cholinesterases in Down syndrome children before and after nutritional supplementation. Singapore Medical Journal. 2008;**49**:561-564

[106] Wiedman AM, Barr SI, Green TJ, Xu Z, Innis SM, Kitts DD. Dietary choline intake: Current state of knowledge across the life cycle. Nutrients. 2018;**10**:1-24. DOI: 10.3390/nu10101513

[107] Powers BE, Kelley CM, Velazquez R, Ash JA, Strawderman MS, Alldred MJ, et al. Maternal choline supplementation in a mouse model of Down syndrome: Effects on attention and nucleus basalis/substantia innominata neuron morphology in adult offspring. Neuroscience. 2017;**340**:501-514. DOI: 10.1016/j.neuroscience.2016.11.001

[108] Ash AS, Velazquez R, Kelley CM, Powers BE, Ginsberg SD, Mufson EJ, et al. Maternal choline supplementation improves spatial mapping and increases basal forebrain cholinergic neuron number and size in aged Ts65Dn mice. Neurobiology of Disease. 2014;**70**:32-42. DOI: 10.1016/j.nbd.2014.06.001

[109] Hijazi M, Fillat C, Medina JM, Velasco A. Overexpression of DYRK1A inhibits choline acetyltransferase induction by oleic acid in cellular models of Down syndrome. Experimental Neurology. 2013;**239**:229-234. DOI: 10.1016/j.expneurol.2012.10.016

[110] Moon J, Chen M, Gandhy SU, Strawderman M, Levitsky DA, Maclean KN, et al. Perinatal choline supplementation improves cognitive functioning and emotion regulation in the Ts65Dn mouse model of Down syndrome. Behavioral Neuroscience. 2010;**124**:346-361. DOI: 10.1037/a0019590

[111] Velazquez R, Ash JA, Powers BE, Kelley CM, Strawderman M, Luscher ZI, et al. Maternal choline supplementation

improves spatial learning and adult hippocampal neurogenesis in the Ts65Dn mouse model of Down syndrome. Neurobiology of Disease. 2013;**58**:92-101. DOI: 10.1016/j.nbd.2013.04.016

[112] Stagni F, Giacomini A, Guidi S, Ciani E, Bartesaghi R. Timing of therapies for Down syndrome: The sooner, the better. Frontiers in Behavioral Neuroscience. 2015;**9**:1-18. DOI: 10.3389/fnbeh.2015.00265

[113] Kleiner G, Barca E, Ziosi M, Emmanuele V, Xu Y, Hidalgo-Gutierrez A, et al. CoQ10 supplementation rescues nephrotic syndrome through normalization of H_2S oxidation pathway. Biochimica et Biophysica Acta, Molecular Basis of Disease. 1864;**2018**:3708-3722. DOI: 10.1016/j.bbadis.2018.09.002

[114] Tiano L, Carnevali P, Padella L, Principi F, Bruge F, Carle F, et al. Effect of Coenzyme Q10 in mitigating oxidative DNA damage in Dpwn syndrome patients, a double blind randomized controlled trial. Neurobiology of Aging. 2011;**32**:2103-2105. DOI: 10.1016/j.neurobiolaging.2009.11.016

[115] Tiano L, Padella L, Santoro L, Carnevali P, Principi F, Brugè F, et al. Prolonged coenzyme Q10 treatment in Down syndrome patients: Effect on DNA oxidation. Neurobiology of Aging. 2012;**33**:626

[116] Larsen EL, Padella L, Morup Bergholdt HK, Henriksen T, Santoro L, Gabrielli O, et al. The effect of long-term treatment with coenzyme Q10 on nucleicacid modifications by oxidation in children with Down syndrome. Neurobiology of Aging. 2018;**67**:159-161. DOI: 10.1016/j.neurobiolaging.2018.03.001

Chapter 3

Impact of Glycine Supplementation to Dietary Crude Protein Reduction in Broiler Chickens

Paschal Chukwudi Aguihe, Ibinabo Imuetinyan Ilaboya and Deji Abiodun Joshua

Abstract

A 21-day experiment was conducted to evaluate the effect of dietary reduction of crude protein (CP) concentrations with graded levels of supplemental glycine (Gly) on growth performance of broiler chickens. Day-old chicks (n = 250) were randomly divided into five treatment groups which were divided into five replicates of ten chicks each in a completely randomized design. The treatments were as follows: T1 comprised of the control group with a standard CP diet (SCPD; 3100 kcal ME/kg and 22% CP) while T2, T3, T4 and T5 comprised of groups fed reduced CP diets (RCPD; 3100 kcal ME/kg and 19% CP) with supplemental Gly at 0.2, 0.4, 0.6 and 0.8% graded levels, respectively. Weight gain (WG), feed intake (FI) and feed conversion ratio (FCR) data was collected on a weekly basis. Final body weight and weight gain of birds fed control and 0.8% Gly diets were similar and higher ($P < 0.05$) than those fed other treatment diets. A similar FCR was recorded among birds fed control, 0.6% and 0.8% Gly diets but lower ($P < 0.05$) than other treatment groups. Therefore, a minimum level of 0.6% Gly supplementation is necessary to optimized performance of broilers (21-d old) fed RCPD.

Keywords: broiler, low protein diet, glycine, performance, glycine supplementation

1. Introduction

The mounting demand of animal proteins for an expanding global population in the face of limited natural resources shall be guided by the responsibility to increase productivity while minimizing environmental impact. Leaving conventional animal feeding methods in the past and shifting to well establish modern dietary strategies could play a substantial role in securing a smaller ecological footprint from animal production. This means lowering dietary crude protein (CP) while supplementing essential amino acids (AA) to cover the nutritional requirements of the broilers. Growing emphasis on environmental regulation requires global animal production to adopt strategies like feeding low CP diets to minimize nitrogen (N) excretion. Furthermore, N excretion declines by approximately 14% providing strong environmental incentives to successfully reducing CP in broiler feeds by greater than 30 g/kg [1–3]. The formulation of these diets is typically based on decreases in soybean meal and increases in feed grain (maize or wheat) contents coupled with elevated inclusions of non-bound (crystalline and synthetic) amino acids to meet requirements. Real benefits for sustainable chicken-meat production using less resources will stem from the successful development of such diets. There is a genuine quest to develop effective, reduced crude protein (CP)-diets for broiler chickens because their acceptance would generate several material advantages. These advantages range from reduced nitrogen and ammonia emissions, improved litter quality and enhanced bird welfare to less undigested protein passing into the hind gut to fuel the proliferation of potential pathogens [4, 5]. Furthermore, a reduction in dietary CP may improve flock health by reducing the risk of necrotic enteritis (NE) caused by the proliferation of *Clostridium perfringens* in the hind gut [6, 7]. The economic benefits of reducing dietary CP stem from reductions in energy expenditure on excreting excess N as uric acid and sparing of matrix space in feed formulation for inclusion of less energy dense ingredients, potentially reducing feed costs [8]. Besides, reducing dietary CP has a particular advantage for producers in tropical and subtropical regions especially sub-sahara Africa; where heat stress is a common problem in poultry production, and causes major economic losses annually [9, 10]. Given the fact that heat increment of CP is the highest, compared to fat and carbohydrates [11], it has been proposed that the adverse effects of heat stress on poultry performance can be alleviated by reducing CP [12, 13].

However, in some of the animal feeding studies, lowering dietary CP beyond a certain level showed undesirable effects on growth performance and carcass quality of broilers [14–17]. Whilst greater reductions of dietary CP (40 to 50 g/kg) invariably compromise broiler performance and increase lipid deposition, a limited number of studies have investigated both aspects [16, 18, 19]. Thus, inferior FCR and increased fat deposition epitomize the challenges to successfully reducing dietary CP using substantial levels of non-bound amino acids. Such findings imply that there is a threshold to CP reductions that can be accommodated by broiler chickens. If the factors contributing to this threshold were to be identified it should be possible to put corrective strategies in place so that tangibly reduced-CP diets, with their attendant advantages, will meet acceptance.

A number of explanatory approaches or reasons have been advanced or debated as the possible consequences of tangibly lowering dietary CP on broiler performance [20]. The difference in the optimal ratio of essential AA between experimental diets [21], specific non-essential AA [22] and utilization of free AA compared to peptide bound AA [16] are among the approaches mostly discussed. Considering the sum of nonessential amino acids probably is not sufficient because specific metabolic processes can become limiting [23]. This leads to the implication that single nonessential amino acids are important to avoid unfavorable effects of low crude protein feed on the growth of broiler chickens [24, 25]. Single nonessential amino acids have been supplemented to low crude protein feed in several studies. Supplementing free glutamic acid, aspartic acid, proline, and alanine consistently did not prevent from reduced growth caused by feeding low crude protein feed [26, 27]. However, growth-increasing effects were determined when free glycine was supplemented. Two studies showed that supplementing feed with a crude protein concentration of 16% with free glycine to the level of about 22% crude protein control feed prevented reduction of growth compared to the control feed [27–29].

However, the concentration of glycine in nutrition of broiler chickens cannot be considered alone because studies revealed that serine in the feed has the same effect on the growth as glycine [30]. Animals can convert glycine into serine and vice versa. On a molar basis, serine is considered to be as effective as Gly for various functions in poultry due to the inter-conversion between the two amino acids [30]. Owing to their assumed unlimited metabolic inter-conversion, Gly and Ser are usually assessed simultaneously when determining the physiological value of diets. Most studies use the sum of both Gly and Ser concentrations, usually termed 'Gly + Ser' to capture the analogous effect of these AAs. Therefore, this study was carried out to evaluate the impact of reducing crude protein concentration with feed-grade glycine supplementation in corn-soybean based diet of broiler chicken on growth performance during the period of 1–21 days of age.

2. Materials and method

2.1 Husbandry and treatments

A total of 250 day old mixed-sex broilers (Arbor acre) with comparable initial body weights were raised at 10 chicks/replicate in a deep litter pens under standard environmental and hygienic practices from day 1 to 35. They were acquired from a reputable commercial hatchery and immunized at the hatchery following a vaccination regime for Arbor acre strain. Birds had free access to mash feed and freshwater during the course of the trial. Feeds (**Table 1**) based on corn and soybean for starter (1–21 days) phase were prepared according to the recent NRC broiler chicken's nutritional requirements except for CP. The experiment was performed as a completely randomized design with five dietary treatments arranged in five replications of 10 chicks each. The treatments were as follows: T1 comprised of the control group with a standard CP diet (SCPD) while T2, T3, T4 and T5 comprised of groups fed reduced CP diets (RCPD) with supplemental Gly at 0.2, 0.4, 0.6 and 0.8% graded levels respectively. Diets (mash) and water were provided ad libitum throughout the experiment. All experimental diets were made isocaloric to contain 3100 kcal ME/kg; whereas, SCPD was formulated to contain 22% CP and the RCPD were isonitrogenous to contain 19% CP for T2 – T5. The feed formulation and nutritional composition of the starter (1–21 days of age) diets are shown in **Table 1**. Dietary treatment groups were set up in an alternating pen pattern within the facility. All birds were housed in the Poultry Research Facility of the Department of Animal Production and Health Technology at the Federal College of Wildlife Management, New Bussa, Niger state, Nigeria. All animals were maintained according to the guidelines specified by the Research Committee Council on Animal Care, and protocols were approved by the Federal College of Wildlife Management Animal Care and Use Committee.

2.2 Sampling and measurements

Body weight (BW) was measured weekly for each pen. Feed intake was determined as the difference between the amount of feed offered and the amount unconsumed in starter and grower phase. The daily feed intake (DFI) was calculated by dividing each pen's consumed feed on starter and grower phase by actual total number of birds. The feed conversion ratio (FCR: g feed/g body weight gain) was calculated by dividing daily feed intake by daily body weight gain. On day 35, two birds per replicate with a BW close to the pen average weight were chosen, and the blood for biochemical analyses was taken from the jugular vein and centrifuged at 3000 rpm for

Ingredients	SCPD[b]	RCPD[c] + 0.2% Gly	RCPD +0.4% Gly	RCPD +0.60%Gly	RCPD +0.80%Gly
Maize	51.19	60.00	60.00	60.00	60.00
Soybean	38.58	30.45	30.45	30.25	30.23
Soya-oil	4.90	4.00	4.00	4.00	3.82
DCP	1.95	2.00	2.00	2.00	2.00
Limestone	1.38	1.40	1.40	1.40	1.40
Salt	0.50	0.50	0.50	0.50	0.50
Premix[a]	0.50	0.50	0.50	0.50	0.50
DL-methionine	0.25	0.30	0.30	0.30	0.30
L-Lysine	0.15	0.30	0.30	0.30	0.30
L-Glycine	0.00	0.20	0.40	0.60	0.80
L-Threonine	0.00	0.15	0.15	0.15	0.15
Inert Filler	0.60	0.20	0.00	0.00	0.00
Total	100	100	100	100	100
Nutrients level					
Crude protein	22.09	19.40	19.40	19.31	19.30
ME[d]	3193.72	3198.15	3198.15	3192.75	3177.09
Lysine	1.12	1.12	1.12	1.12	1.12
Methionine	0.56	0.59	0.59	0.59	0.59
Cystine	0.30	0.28	0.28	0.28	0.28
Met+Cys	0.85	0.87	0.87	0.86	0.86
Threonine	0.90	0.93	0.93	0.93	0.93
Arginine	1.27	1.10	1.10	1.09	1.09
Isoleucine	0.94	0.82	0.82	0.82	0.82
Leucine	1.92	1.81	1.81	1.80	1.80
Valine	0.97	0.87	0.87	0.86	0.86
Histidine	0.97	0.83	0.83	0.82	0.82
Phenylalanine	1.13	1.01	1.01	1.01	1.01
Glycine	0.90	0.99	1.18	1.37	1.56
Serine	1.13	1.00	1.00	1.00	0.99
Gly + Ser	2.03	1.98	2.18	2.36	2.56

[a]Vitamin/Mineral Premix supplied per kg of the diet: Vit A: 10,000iu; Vit D: 28000iu; Vit E: 35,000iu; Vit K: 1900 mg; Vit B12: 19 mg; Riboflavin: 7000 mg; Pyridoxine: 3800 mg; Thiamine: 2200 mg; Pantothenic acid: 11000 mg; Nicotinic acid: 45,000 mg; Folic acid: 1400 mg; Biotin: 113 mg; Cu: 8000 mg; Mn: 64000 mg; Zn: 40, 000 mg; Fe: 32000 mg; Se: 160 mg; Iodine: 800 mg; Cobalt: 400 mg; Choline: 475000 mg.
[b]SCPD: Standard crude protein diet.
[c]RCPD: Reduced crude protein diet.
[d]ME: Metabolizable energy.

Table 1.
Ingredients composition and nutrient levels of experimental diets (% as fed).

10 min to separate serum that was stored at -80°C. The serum concentrations of total protein, albumin, glucose, triglyceride, and creatinine were determined by utilizing enzymatic colorimetric kits as specified by the manufacturer. Serum globulin was estimated accordingly by subtracting albumin from total protein.

2.3 Statistical analysis

The statistical processing of the results was done using general linear model (GLM) of SPSS, version 20.0 (SPSS Inc., Chicago, IL, USA). When comparing treatments means, post hoc Tukey's multiple range test was carried out to assess any significant differences for the measured parameters. Differences were considered significant at $p < .05$. Replicate-pen was used as the experimental units for the analysis.

3. Result and discussion

Growth performance of the broiler chicks fed RCPD containing graded levels of supplemental glycine are shown in **Table 2**. At day 21, the results of the present study showed that glycine supplementation did not affect ($P > 0.05$) the initial body weight and feed intake, however, significant differences ($P < 0.05$) were observed on final body weight, weight gain and FCR of the broiler chicks. Chicks fed control diet had higher ($p < 0.05$) final body weight and weight gain than the chicks fed RCPD with 0.2, 0.4 and 0.6% supplemental glycine levels. Similar ($p > 0.05$) final body weight and weight gain were observed among chicks fed control diet and 0.8% Gly supplemented RCPD. Birds fed control, 0.6 and 0.8% Gly diets have similar ($p > 0.05$) feed conversion ratio, and were lower ($p < 0.05$) than those on RCPD with 0.2 and

Treatment	Initial weight (g/bird)	Final body weight (g/bird)	Feed intake (g/bird)	Weight gain (g/bird)	FCR
T1	42.54	893.26^{a}	1111.67	850.72^{a}	1.31^{a}
T2	42.73	723.87^{d}	1195.63	681.14^{d}	1.76^{a}
T3	42.89	794.11^{c}	1164.75	751.22^{c}	1.55^{b}
T4	42.58	825.14^{b}	1156.63	782.56^{b}	1.48^{ab}
T5	42.55	871.82^{a}	1148.22	829.27^{a}	1.38^{a}
SEM	1.65	12.12	25.86	10.93	0.08
p-values	0.141	0.032	0.311	0.016	0.002

[a]*Means within column with no common superscripts differ significantly ($p < 0.05$).*
[b]*Means within column with no common superscripts differ significantly ($p < 0.05$).*
[c]*Means within column with no common superscripts differ significantly ($p < 0.05$).*
[d]*Means within column with no common superscripts differ significantly ($p < 0.05$).*
T1: Standard crude protein diet (Control).
T2: Reduced crude protein diet +0.2% glycine.
T3: Reduced crude protein diet +0.4% glycine.
T4: Reduced crude protein diet +0.6% glycine.
T5: Reduced crude protein diet +0.8% glycine.
SEM: Standard Error Mean.

Table 2.
Growth performance of broiler chicken (1–21 d old) fed reduced crude protein diets with graded levels of supplemental glycine.

0.4% Gly diet. The present study showed that increasing levels of supplemental Gly increased weight gain and decreased feed conversion ratio among the experimental birds. Gly addition at 0.2 and 0.4% levels which provided 1.98 and 2.18% total Gly + Ser, respectively in the diets failed to completely overcome the adverse impact of dietary reduction of CP by 3% on the performance of the broiler chickens at 21 d old. This observation corroborates with the findings of Awad et al. [30] who concluded that the provision of 2.02–2.22% dietary Gly + Ser during starter period failed to support optimal growth performance in broiler chickens raised under tropical climate. However, providing 2.36 and 2.56% total Gly + Ser concentration in the RCPD through increased supplementation of Gly at 0.6 and 0.8% levels were observed to restored the FCR to equal those group fed control diet.

This present finding is in agreement with the reports of previous researchers [18, 27, 31, 32] who confirmed that maintaining a minimum level of 2.32% in diets via Gly supplementation allowed to decreased dietary CP concentration up to 3% or more without compromising the accumulative growth performance of broiler chickens (1–21 d old). Also, our result is in accordance with previous reports which suggested that maintenance of optimal amino acid ratios for essential amino acids and sufficient total Gly + Ser levels appear most important considerations in formulating broiler diets with reduced CP concentrations [2, 25, 33–35]. According to Kamely et al. [35], feeding low protein diets formulated to provide higher Gly + Ser and meet digestible amino acid requirements could be an efficient way to reduce nitrogen excretion to the environment and decrease feed cost without impacting growth performance. Also, the current result concur with the report of Siegert et al. [22], who conducted a meta-analysis of 10 studies and concluded that sufficient supply of dietary Gly + Ser had significant positive effects on weight gain and feed conversion efficiency of birds fed low CP diets. Understanding the active roles play by Gly in several number of non-protein pathways can further account for the reasons why it can potentially improve the performance of broiler chickens supplied with RCPD [36, 37]. Gly plays significant function for methionine recycling and cysteine biosynthesis, threonine catabolism, uric acid and creatine synthesis [38]. Moreover, Gly represents the main part of the gut mucin glycoproteins [39]. In essence, Gly can promote the metabolic and nutritional efficiency of EAA as well as gut functionality and consequently growth performance [13, 40, 41]. In view of these key metabolic roles of Gly, although it is notionally a non-essential amino acid; Gly may become conditionally limiting in reduced CP diets formulated based on vegetable ingredients [41–43]. Provision of higher dietary level of Gly + Ser via increased Gly supplementation may be essential to achieve greater CP reduction without compromising the growth performance of growing broiler chickens [13, 32, 40].

4. Conclusion and recommendation

In the present study, increasing dietary levels of glycine supplementation resulted in an increased body weight gain and improved feed conversion ratio of broiler chicks fed diets containing reduced crude protein concentration. Maintaining a minimum of 0.6% supplemental Gly that provided 2.36% Gly + Ser level has shown to support the reduction of crude protein concentration from 22 to 19% in diet of broiler chickens at 21 days of age, without undermining their accumulative growth performance and concomitantly minimizing the impact of broiler production on the environment. Therefore, higher Gly supplementation (0.6–0.8% inclusion) can be recommended for the initial stages of growth of broiler chickens up to 21 d of age, based on weight gain and feed conversion responses raised under tropical environment.

As Gly have the potential to limit growth performance of broiler chickens, this amino acid, ideally on a digestible basis, should appear in recommendations suitable for facilitating low CP diets, because such diets are expected to become more important in the future. Growing evidence in the present study shows that a sufficient provision of supplemental glycine is necessary for the optimal growth of chickens. Thus, ideal protein diets for poultry must supply all physiologically and nutritionally amino acids to maximize their growth performance and productivity. This nutritional strategy is expected to facilitate the formulation of low-protein diets and precision nutrition through the addition of low-cost supplemental amino acids or their alternative sources of animal proteins. In regions where free crystalline glycine is prohibited or not approved, an adequate dietary Gly + Ser supply can only be achieved by inclusion of feedstuffs of animal origin which represent good source of glycine, to prepare balanced low protein diets for chickens and help sustain the global animal agriculture for increased food productivity. Thus, in our study, dietary crude protein was reduced with supplemental glycine fortification up to 3% without any adverse effects on broiler performance. So, in future, when amino acid industry expanded and all nutritional amino acids distributed as feed grade supplements for animal use, it could be possible reduce crude protein up to 6% which will be more economic. If progress in these directions can be actualized, then the prospects of reduced protein diets contributing to sustainable chicken-meat production are promising and becomes increasingly real.

Acknowledgements

The authors wish to acknowledge the support of the management of Federal College of Wildlife Management, New Bussa, Nigeria, towards the success of this research project.

Conflict of interest

The authors declare that they have no conflicts of interest associated with this manuscripts.

Author details

Paschal Chukwudi Aguihe[1*], Ibinabo Imuetinyan Ilaboya[2] and Deji Abiodun Joshua[3]

1 Department of Animal Production Technology, Federal College of Wildlife Management, New Bussa, Nigeria

2 Department of Animal Science, Benson Idahosa University, Benin, Nigeria

3 Department of Basic Science, Federal College of Wildlife Management, New Bussa, Nigeria

*Address all correspondence to: aguihepc@gmail.com

References

[1] Kriseldi R, Tillman PB, Jiang Z, Dozier WA III. Effects of feeding reduced crude protein diets on growth performance, nitrogen excretion, and plasma uric acid concentration of broiler chicks during the starter period. Poultry Science. 2018;**97**:1614-1626

[2] Chrystal PV, Moss AF, Khoddami A, Naranjo VD, Selle PH, Liu SY. Impacts of reduced-crude protein diets on key parameters in male broiler chickens offered maize-based diets. Poultry Science. 2020;**99**:505-516. DOI: 10.3382/ps/pez573

[3] Van Harn J, Dijkslag MA, Van Krimpen M. Effect of low protein diets supplemented with free amino acids on growth performance, slaughter yield, litter quality, and footpad lesions of male broilers. Poultry Science. 2019;**1**:e10

[4] Garland PW. The challenges confronting chicken meat producers in Great Britain in relation to low protein diets. Australian Poultry Science Symp. 2018;**29**(1):e7

[5] Lemme A, Hiller P, Klahsen M, Taube V, Stegemann J, Simon I. Reduction of dietary protein in broiler diets not only reduces n-emissions but is also accompanied by several further benefits. Journal of Applied Poultry Research. 2019;**28**:867-880. DOI: 10.3382/japr/pfz045

[6] Drew MD, Syed NA, Goldade BG, Laarveld B, Van Kessel AG. Effects of dietary protein source and level on intestinal populations of *Clostridium perfringens* in broiler chickens. Poultry Science. 2004;**83**(414):e20

[7] Wilkie DC, van Kessel AG, White LJ, Laarveld B, Drew MD. Dietary amino acids affectintestinal Clostridium perfringens populations in broiler chickens. Canadian. Journal of Animal Science. 2005;**85, 185**:e93

[8] Liu SY, Macelline SP, Chrystal PV, Selle PH. Progress towards reduced-crude protein diets for broiler chickens and sustainable chicken-meat production. Journal of Animal Science and Biotechnology. 2021;**12**:20-33

[9] Daghir NJ. Poultry Production in Hot Climates. Wallinford, UK: CAB International; 2008

[10] Lara LJ, Rostagno MH. Impact of heat stress on poultry production. Animals. 2013;**3**:356-369

[11] Musharaf NA, Latshaw JD. Heat increment as affected by protein and amino acid nutrition. World's Poultry Science Journal. 1999;**55**:233-240

[12] Zaman QU, Mushtaq T, Nawaz H, Mirza MA, Mahmood S, Ahmad T, et al. Effect of varying dietary energy and protein on broiler performance in hot climate. Animal Feed Science and Technology. 2008;**146**:302-312

[13] Namroud NF, Shivazad M, Zaghari M. Effects of fortifying low crude protein diet with crystalline amino acids on performance, blood ammonia level, and excreta characteristics of broiler chicks. Poultry Science. 2008;**87**:2250-2258

[14] Yang H, Yang Z, Wang Z, Wang W, Huang K, Fan W, et al. Effects of early dietary energy and protein dilution on growth performance, nutrient utilization and internal organs of broilers. Italian Journal of Anima Science. 2015;**14**:e3729

[15] Chrystal PV, Greenhalgh S, Selle PH, Liu SY. Facilitating the acceptance of tangibly reduced-crude protein diets for chicken-meat production. Animal Nutrition. 2020;**6**:247-257

[16] Macelline SP, Chrystal PV, Liu SY, Selle PH. Implications of elevated threonine plasma concentrations in the development of reduced-crude protein diets for broiler chickens. Animal Production Science. 2021;**61**:1442-1448

[17] Wang WW, Wang J, Wu SG, Zhang HJ, Qi GH. Response of broilers to gradual dietary protein reduction with or without an adequate glycine plus serine level. Italian Journal of Animal Science. 2020;**19**(1):127-136

[18] Hilliar M, Hargreave G, Girish CK, Barekatain R, Wu SB, Swick RA. Using crystalline amino acids to supplement broiler chicken requirements in reduced protein diets. Poultry Science 2020;**99**:1551-1563. DOI: 10.1016/j.psj.2019.12.005

[19] Aftab U, Ashraf M, Jiang Z. Low protein diets for broilers. World's Poultry Science Journal. 2006;**62**:688-701

[20] Kobayashi H, Nakashima K, Ishida A, Ashihara A, Katsumata M. Effects of low protein diet and low protein diet supplemented with synthetic essential amino acids on meat quality of broiler chickens. Animal Science Journal. 2013;**84**(6):489-495. DOI: 10.1111/asj.12021

[21] Corzo A, Kidd MT, Burnham DJ, Kerr BJ. Dietary glycine needs of broiler chicks. Poultry Science. 2004;**83**:1382-1384

[22] Siegert W, Ahmadi H, Rodehutscord M. Meta-analysis of the influence of dietary glycine and serine, with consideration of methionine and cysteine, on growth and feed conversion of broilers. Poultry Science. 2015;**94**(1853):e63

[23] Waldroup PW. Do crude protein levels really matter? In: Proc. 15th Annual ASAIM Southeast Asian Feed Technology and Nutrition Workshop. Conrad Bali Resort, Indonesia; 2007. pp. 1-5

[24] Chrystal PV, Moss AF, Yin D, Khoddami A, Naranjo VD, Selle PH, et al. Glycine equivalent and threonine inclusions in reduced-crude protein, maize-based diets impact on growth performance, fat deposition, starch-protein digestive dynamics and amino acid metabolism in broiler chickens. Animal Feed Science and Technology. 2020;**261**(114837):1e14

[25] Saleh AA, Amber KA, Soliman MM, Soliman MY, Morsy WA, Shukry M, et al. Effect of low protein diets with amino acids supplementation on growth performance, carcass traits, blood parameters and muscle amino acids profile in broiler chickens under high ambient temperature. Agriculture. 2021;**11**:185-197

[26] Dean DW, Bidner TD, Southern LL. Glycine supplementation to low protein, amino acid supplemented diets supports optimal performance of broiler chicks. Poultry Science. 2006;**85**(288):e96

[27] Awad EA, Zulkifli I, Soleimani AF, Loh TC. Individual non-essential amino acids fortification of a low-protein diet for broilers under the hot and humid tropical climate. Poultry Science. 2015;**94**:2772-2777

[28] Baghban-Kanani P, Azimi-Youvalari S. Interactive effects of glycine and threonine in low protein broiler diets on performance, blood ammonia level, intestinal mucosa development

and nutrient digestibility. Acta Scientific Veterinary Sciences. 2022;**4**(1):1-2

[29] Sugahara M, Kandatsu M. Glycine serine inter-conversion in the rooster. Agricultural and Biological Chemistry. 1976;**40**:833-837

[30] Awad EA, Zulkifli I, Soleimani AF, Aljuobori A. Effects of feeding male and female broiler chickens on low-protein diets fortified with different dietary glycine levels under the hot and humid tropical climate. Italian Journal of Animal Science. 2017;**16**:453-461

[31] Aguihe PC, Ospina-Rojas IC, Sakamoto MI, Pozza PC, Iyayi EA, Murakami AE. Dietary glycine equivalent and standardized ileal digestible methionine + cysteine levels for male broiler chickens fed low-crude-protein diets. Canadian Journal of Animal Science. 2022;**102**(1):19-29. DOI: 10.1139/CJAS-2021-0009

[32] Lemme A, Hiller P, Klahsen M, Taube V, Stegemann J, Simon I. Reduction of dietary proteinin broiler diets not only reduces n-emissions but is also accompanied by several further benefits. Journal of Applied Poultry Research. 2019;**28**:867-880. DOI: 10.3382/japr/pfz045

[33] Hofmann P, Siegert W, Kenéz Á, Naranjo VD, Rodehutscord M. Very low crude protein and varying glycine concentrations in the diet affect growth performance, characteristics of nitrogen excretion, and the blood metabolome of broiler chickens. Journal of Nutrition. 2019;**149**:1122-1132. DOI: 10.1093/jn/nxz022

[34] Aguihe PC, Hirata KA, Ospina-Rojas CI, dos Santos TC, Pozza PC, Iyayi EA, et al. Effect of glycine equivalent levels in low protein diet containing different SID threonine concentrations on performance, serum metabolites and muscle creatine of broiler chickens. Italian Journal of Animal Science. 2022;**21**(1):1000-1009

[35] Kamely M, He W, Wakaruk J, Whelan R, Naranjo V, Barreda DR. Impact of reduced dietary crude protein in the starter phase on immune development and response of broilers throughout the growth period. Frontiers in Veterinary Science. 2020;**7**:436-449. DOI: 10.3389/fvets.2020.00436

[36] Akinde DO. Amino acid efficiency with dietary glycine supplementation: Part 1. World's Poultry Science Journal. 2014;**70**:461-474

[37] Akinde DO. Amino acid efficiency with dietary glycine supplementation: Part 2. World's Poultry Science Journal. 2014;**70**:575-584

[38] Hejdysz M, Bogucka J, Ziółkowska E, Perz K, Jarosz L, Ciszewski A, et al. Effects of low crude protein content and glycine supplementation on broiler chicken performance, carcass traits, and litter quality. Livestock Science. 2022;**261**:104930. DOI: 10.1016/j.livsci.2022.104930

[39] Ospina-Rojas IC, Murakami AE, Eyng C, Nunes RV, Duarte CRA, Vargas MD. Commercially available amino acid supplementation of low-protein diets for broiler chickens with different ratios of digestible glycine+serine: Lysine. Poultry Science. 2012;**91**:3148-3155. DOI: 10.3382/ps.2012-02470

[40] Ospina-Rojas IC, Murakami AE, Moreira I, Picoli KP, Rodrigueiro RJB, Furlan AC. Dietary glycine+serine responses of male broilers given low-protein diets with different concentrations of threonine. British Poultry Science. 2013;**54**:486-493

[41] Siegert W, Wild KJ, Schollenberger M, Helmbrecht A, Rodehutscord M. Effect of glycine supplementation in low protein diets with amino acids from soy protein isolate or free amino acids on broiler growth and nitrogen utilization. British Poultry Science. 2016;**57**(424):e34

[42] Hilliar M, Morgan N, Hargreave G, Barekatain R, Wu S, Swick R. Glycine supplementationof low protein diets in broilers. Aus Poul Sci Symp. 2017;**28**:158

[43] Kriseldi R, Tillman PB, Jiang Z, Dozier WA III. Effects of glycine and glutamine supplementation to reduced crude protein diets on growth performance and carcass characteristics of male broilers during a 41-day production period. Journal of Applied Poultry Research. 2017;**26**(558):e72

Chapter 4

DHA (Docosahexaenoic Acid): A Biomolecule with Diverse Roles and Health Benefits

Abdul Hei and Laishram Sanahanbi

Abstract

With the increasing interest in health and nutrition for longevity of life and more performance ability, the idea of health foods and nutrients has attracted more research and studies. Omega-3 fatty acid docosahexaenoic acid (DHA) is a nutrient molecule with various diverse roles and health benefits in the human body. Though DHA originally comes from microalgae and sea plants, the main source of DHA is fish, shellfish, and fish oils. DHA is a key nutrient with a structural and functional role in the cell membrane and cell organelles, and abundant in brain and eye. It is good for the heart, and protective against heart diseases. It is rather a very ancient molecule with more modern concepts. Really, DHA has been proven to be a key nutrient that is required in the processes of physical and mental development and health, and prevention of diseases throughout the life span. Driven by the values of physical and mental health, the demand for DHA in the international market is expected to grow. This review is an attempt to update the research findings about DHA and its health benefits in an easy and lucid way.

Keywords: DHA, fish oils, diseases prevention, health, more ability

1. Introduction

Everybody on this planet would like to lead a beautiful, happy, and meaningful life. However, we are what we eat. A sound body and a sound mind come from what we are made up of. So, a perfect knowledge of what we intake daily in our diet and especially in the stages of pregnancy, infancy, and childhood is very important. Interest in omega-3 fatty acids has increased in recent years because of their various roles in health promotion and disease risk reduction [1]. With increasing interest in health consciousness and our well-being, the essential omega-3 fatty acids have been the most studied biomolecules during the last few decades. These omega-3 fatty acids have strong implications in medicine as they have been linked to various health conditions, such as inflammation, cancer, heart diseases, and neurological disorders. Docosahexaenoic acid DHA is the key component of all cell membranes of the body and the most important fatty acid, which is concentrated in the brain and central nervous system and is referred to as "brain food." On account of its diverse amazing roles and health benefit, it has become the star nutrient molecule nowadays [2]. Bradburry call the DHA molecule an ancient molecule for the modern human brain [3].

An optimum level of the omega-3 fatty acid DHA in the body is required for efficient body functions. Omega-3 fatty acids have been linked to healthy aging throughout life [4]. As these PUFA are essential, normal infant/neonatal brain, intellectual growth, and development cannot be accomplished if they are deficient during pregnancy and lactation. Sustaining normal adult brain function also requires PUFA.

Studies suggest that the evolution of large human brain occurred depending on the rich source of preformed long-chain PUFA at the interface of land and water. The human diet has changed to a large extent during the last 100 years. One of the striking changes is the enormous increase in dietary fat. In terms of quality, we have increased our intakes of saturated fatty acids (SFA), alpha-linoleic acid (LA) and *trans* fatty acids, concomitant with reduced intakes of (n-3) fatty acids. The latter comprises reduced intake of 3-linolenic acid (ALA) rich foods, and less consumption of long-chain PUFA of the (n-3) series [LC(n-3)P], that is, eicosapentaenoic (EPA) and docosahexaenoic (DHA) acids notably from fish [1]. These dietary and other environmental changes are deemed to be among the major causes of the rapid expansion of diet-related chronic disease [2], including cardiovascular disease (CVD) in the past century [5].

The question is: Are we getting enough of the DHA in our daily diet? DHA is found mainly in seafood, such as fish, shellfish, and fish oils. It is also found in some types of algae [6]. So, the objective of the chapter is to review and discuss the diverse amazing health benefits and roles and to make sure if we are getting enough DHA in our diet.

2. Defining DHA: one biomolecule diverse functions

DHA (docosahexaenoic acid) is an important omega -3 polyunsaturated fatty acid (PUFA) consisting of a long chain of 22 carbon atoms and 6 double bonds. DHA is mainly found in fish and fish oil with EPA. It is remarkable that one simple molecule has been reported to affect so many apparently unrelated biological processes.

DHA molecule is an integral part of all cell membranes and critical to membrane fluidity [7]. Aptly referring to "DHA as brain food," docosahexaenoic acid (DHA) is the predominant omega-3 (n-3) polyunsaturated fatty (PUFA) found in the brain and can do neurological function through signal transduction, pathway, neurotransmission, neurogenesis, membrane receptor function, synaptic plasticity, healthy inflammation balance, membrane organization, and membrane integrity [8].

Important functions of DHA include antioxidant activity, memory formation, neurogenesis, acting as a signaling molecule. Researchers conclude that it is fairly astonishing how DHA, a single molecule, plays so many roles. The present-day diet typically lacks appreciable amounts of DHA. Therefore, in modern population maintaining optimal levels of DHA in the brain throughout the lifespan likely requires obtaining preformed DHA *via* dietary supplemental sources. Most omega-3 supplements contain both DHA and EPA but there are many high-quality DHA supplements also available when more of this precious nutrient is desirable.

3. Sources of DHA

Important omega-3 fatty acids are DHA, EPA, and ALA. Polyunsaturated fatty acids, particularly n-3 PUFA, DHA, and EPA are the prominent compounds found in fish [9]. ALA is present in different plant seeds and grains that convert a small amount into EPA and DHA after human consumption. Flaxseed oil is a major plant source of ALA [10]. In the human diet, the main contributors of DHA and EPA are marine ecosystems (fish, shellfish, and other sea foods) [11]. Fish liver contains a large number of omega-3 fatty acids that have been proven by different studies to lower blood triglycerides and cholesterol levels. Actually, fatty predatory fish like sharks have a lot of omega-3 fatty acids in their tissues that possess a lot of health benefits, particularly in terms of reducing inflammation, improving mental health, and serving as an antioxidant [11]. Fatty fishes, such as *Salmo salar* (salmon *Gadus morhua* (cod), *Thunnus thynnus* (tuna),) *Tenualosa ilisha, Sardinella longiceps, Schizothorax richardsonii*, and *Neolisochilus hexaganolepis,* have numerous roles as main sources of DHA and other polyunsaturated fatty acids [12]. Micro- and macroalgae are original sources of DHA [13]. Another study stated that egg yolk contains ALA (0.8%), DHA (0.7%), and EPA (0.1%). Additionally, egg yolk, lean red meat, chicken, and human milk are also good sources of ALA [14].

4. Reason for intake of DHA in our diet

Human body cannot synthesize enough amount of DHA from α-linolenic acid (ALA), under the actions of fatty acid elongases and desaturases, the bioconversion rate in the human body is extremely low, generally at 2–10%), and sometimes, it was reported even at a lower rate of 0.01%. Therefore, DHA-rich or fortified foods and DHA supplements are the two main exogenous sources to obtain additional DHA needed for the biological functions of human body [15].

Important roles of DHA are found in **Figure 1.**

1. Eyes, 2. Brain, 3. Heart, 4. Developing infants and children, 5. Bones, 6. Joints, 7. Skin, and 8. Spermatozoa (**Figure 1**).

Docosahexaenoic acid (DHA) is essential for the growth and functional development of the brain in infants. DHA is also needed for the maintenance of normal brain function in adults. The inclusion of plentiful DHA in the diet boosts learning ability,

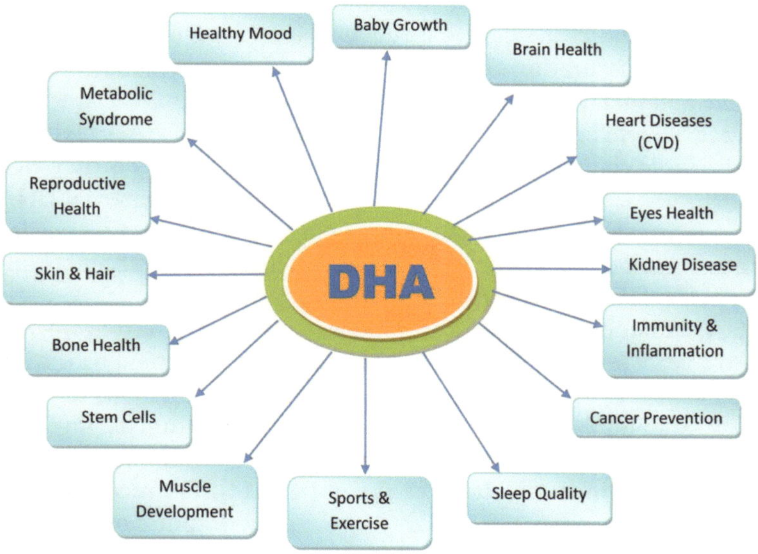

Figure 1.
Picture showing important benefits of DHA.

whereas deficiencies of DHA are associated with deficits in learning. DHA deficiencies are also associated with fetal alcohol syndrome, attention deficit hyperactivity disorder, cystic fibrosis, phenylketonuria, unipolar depression, aggressive hostility, and adrenoleukodystrophy [16]. Decreases in DHA in the brain are correlated with cognitive decline during aging and with the onset of sporadic Alzheimer's disease.

Several researchers have shown that ω-3 PUFAs play a major role in altering blood lipid profiles and membrane lipid composition and affect eicosanoid biosynthesis, cell signaling cascades, and gene expression, thereby influencing health [17, 18]. In addition, the beneficial effect of ω-3 PUFAs in patients with myriad health conditions and diseases, such as cardiovascular disease (atrial fibrillation, atherosclerosis, thrombosis, inflammation, and sudden cardiac death, among others), diabetes, cancer, depression and various mental illnesses, age-related cognitive decline, periodontal disease, and rheumatoid arthritis, has been investigated [19, 20].

5. Brain development during pregnancy and early life

Controlling and shaping a child's destiny should start from the stage of pregnancy. Nutrition in pregnancy, during lactation, childhood, and later stages has an important influence on overall development. DHA is a bioactive omega-3 polyunsaturated fatty acid that influences membrane structure and function, cell signaling and communication mechanisms, gene expression, and lipid mediator production. DHA is found in high concentrations in the human brain and eye, where it is linked to better development and function. Maintenance of DHA concentration is important throughout the life course, but pregnancy, lactation, and infancy are vulnerable periods, whereas insufficient DHA supply can impact mental and visual development and performance [21].

Docosahexaenoic acid, 22:6n-3 (DHA), is crucially necessary for the structure and development of the growing fetal brain in utero. DHA is the dominant n-3 long-chain polyunsaturated fatty acid in brain gray matter representing about 15% of all fatty acids in the human frontal cortex. DHA has roles in neurogenesis, neurotransmitter, synaptic plasticity and transmission, and signal transduction in the brain. Data from human and animal studies indicate that adequate levels of DHA in neural membranes are required for the maturation of cortical astrocyte, neurovascular coupling, and glucose uptake and metabolism. Besides, some metabolites of DHA are protective against oxidative tissue injury and stress in the brain. A low DHA level in the brain produces behavioral changes and is associated well with learning difficulties and dementia. In humans, the third trimester-placental supply of maternal DHA to the growing fetus is crucially important as the growing brain obligatorily needs DHA during this window period. Moreover, DHA takes part in the early placentation process, essential for placental development [22].

Docosahexaenoic acid has a rapid accumulation in the brain from week 30 of pregnancy to 2 years postpartum. About 67 mg of DHA is accrued by the fetus per day, thereby increasing its brain weight and making it important for the mother to have adequate DHA intake during this time. The DHA accretion during lactation is 70–80 mg/day, and this huge demand for DHA during lactation depletes maternal stores and may take months to recover even partially [14]. The increasing concentration of DHA takes place nearly 30-fold during the growth spurts of the brain, which corresponds to the beginning of the third trimester of pregnancy to 18 months after birth [23]. During these early growth spurts, the brain is critically vulnerable to nutritional deficiencies. Preterm infants much miss out on the chance of DHA accretion during the last trimester and thus would benefit from external supplementation [24]. Arachidonic acid begins accretion in the brain during the last trimester of pregnancy and continues to accumulate until 2 years of postnatal age. Accretion of about 95 mg/day of ARA takes place during the last 5 weeks of gestation; this is nearly twice the amount of DHA accrued during the same period. A larger amount of the ARA is accumulated in the adipose tissue and skeletal muscles, with relatively lesser amounts accumulated in the brain [25].

A supply of DHA is very important early in life, especially during the fetal and early infant periods when the eye and central nervous system are developing. During pregnancy, transfer of DHA including EPA is done through the placenta from mother to the fetus [26]. The level of omega-3 fatty acid in the fetus is correlated with the amount ingested by the mother, so it is essential that the mother has adequate nutrition [4]. The function of DHA in the brain is to support the transmission of messages through nerve cells and to protect the brain against the loss of scaffolding proteins and oxidative degradation of lipids, thus helping maintain the plasticity of the brain [27]. DHA also plays a functional role in gene expression, myelination, and growth and differentiation of neurons [28]. DHA is also a basic membrane component of the photoreceptor cells of the eye, and proper functioning of the photoreceptor cells is essential for vision [29, 30]. Arachidonic acid is an omega-6 (n-6) fatty acid that plays important roles in brain functioning, including neuronal firing, signal transmission, and long-term potentiation. Besides, ARA preserves hippocampal neuron membrane plasticity, protects the brain against oxidative stress, and aids in the synthesis of new proteins in brain tissues [31].

EPA and DHA supplementation during pregnancy has been found with multiple benefits for the infant. Numerous studies confirmed the benefit of omega-3 supplementation during pregnancy in terms of proper development of the brain and retina. Of the two most important long-chain omega-3 fatty acids, EPA and DHA, DHA is the more crucial for proper cell membrane function and is vital to the development of the fetal brain and retina [32].

6. DHA supplementation after birth

The need for adequate DHA intake for women does not stop after the birth of a healthy baby. DHA goes on rapidly to accumulate in the brains of infants and young children through at least the second year of life [33]. However, human infants can only synthesize DHA in very limited amount, making them dependent on dietary sources, such as breast milk, formula, or DHA supplements [34].

It has long been known that breastfed infants have higher IQs and more advanced cognition than bottle-fed babies [35, 36]. It is now clearly known that one reason for this difference may be that breast milk normally contains DHA. Like the placenta, the milk-producing apparatus in the human breast routinely pulls DHA and other brain-nourishing fatty acids from the mother's blood in preference to other fats, delivering the highest possible amounts to the breastfed infant. Again, this result can come at the expense of the mother's own DHA supplies if steady intake is not assured. The DHA content of the maternal diet is the most important factor determining how much DHA is found in breast milk. Some experts have raised concerns that the consumption of otherwise healthy low-fat diets by women of reproductive age could reduce the amount of DHA available to them during pregnancy and lactation [37]. Given the known low levels of DHA in most women's diets, this observation strongly suggests that DHA supplementation in nursing mothers is critical to optimizing brain development in their infants. DHA supplementation by nursing mothers increases the DHA content in their milk and in infant red blood cells, which is associated with enhanced visual acuity at 4 months [38, 39] and early language development in breastfed infants [33]. High maternal DHA intake is also associated with improved long-term growth in breastfed children [40–42]. Longer duration of breastfeeding and higher ratios of DHA to arachidonic acid (a precursor to DHA) was associated with higher total IQ scores in these school-aged children. The DHA that gets stored in the brain during infancy is an essential building block for children's cognitive, social, emotional, and behavioral development. Higher levels of DHA in infants are connected to stronger development of language, cognition, social, and motor skills as they move out of infancy and into young childhood [32].

7. DHA and inflammation

The role of omega-3 (EPA + DHA) in promoting the resolution of inflammation is an exciting development. Immunity, inflammation, and metabolic health are interrelated. Inflammation drives poor metabolic health. Inflammation leads to morbidity and mortality. Specific nutritional strategies can target inflammation to improve metabolic health. These same strategies target immunity—P.C. Calder.

Inflammation is a key component of normal host defense mechanisms initiating the immune response and later playing a role in tissue repair. Inappropriate, excessive, or uncontrolled inflammation contributes to human diseases and is believed to play a central role in many of the chronic diseases that characterize modern society [43–45].

Fatty acids can give influence on inflammation through a variety of mechanisms, including acting *via* cell surface and intracellular receptors/sensors that control inflammatory cell signaling and gene expression patterns. Some effects of fatty acids on inflammatory cells seem to be mediated by, or at least are associated with, changes in the fatty acid composition of cell membranes. Alterations in these compositions can modify membrane fluidity, lipid raft formation, cell signaling leading to altered gene expression, and the pattern of lipid and peptide mediator production [43, 45]. Cells within the inflammatory response are typically rich in the n-6 fatty acid arachidonic acid, but the contents of arachidonic acid and of the n-3 fatty acids eicosapentaenoic acid (EPA) and docosahexaenoic acid (DHA) can be altered through oral administration of EPA and DHA. Eicosanoids produced from arachidonic acid have inflammatory roles [45, 46]. EPA also produces eicosanoids and these may have differing properties from those of arachidonic acid-derived eicosanoids. EPA and DHA produce resolvins that are anti-inflammatory and inflammation-resolving. Thus, fatty acid exposure and the fatty acid composition of human inflammatory cells have an impact on their function. As a result of their anti-inflammatory actions, marine n-3 fatty acids have healing roles in rheumatoid arthritis, although benefits in other inflammatory diseases and conditions have not been unequivocally demonstrated [45, 46]. The anti-inflammatory effects of marine n-3 fatty acids may contribute to their protective roles toward atherosclerosis, plaque rupture, and cardiovascular mortality. The role of resolvins and related compounds may be very important because the resolution of inflammation is important in shutting off the ongoing inflammatory process and in limiting tissue damage [44]. Human trials show the benefits of oral n-3 fatty acids in rheumatoid arthritis and in stabilizing advanced atherosclerotic plaques. Intravenous n-3 fatty acids may be useful in critically ill patients through reduced inflammation. The anti-inflammatory and inflammation-resolving actions of EPA, DHA, and their derivatives are of clinical relevance [47].

Evidence suggests that, in addition to the amount of fat, the types of fats consumed can have a differential impact on human health. Their results on the risk of cardiovascular disease have dominated the rationale for these recommendations for the past 50 years [48]. There is increasing recognition by leaders in the nutrition and health field that dietary fats can affect host inflammatory responses [15].

8. DHA and cardiovascular disease

CVD is the leading cause of mortality in the world. For example, the prevalence of CVD in China is still rising [49] and India has a much higher rate of 272 per 10,000 higher than that of the global average of 235 [50]. AHA 2022 reports that CVD is the leading cause of death in America [7]. Some researchers have shown that n-3 fatty acids play a role in the protection against cardiovascular heart disease [51], sudden coronary death [52, 53], and peripheral arterial disease [54]. In addition, n- 3 omega-3 fatty acids have multiple beneficial effects on reducing cardio-metabolic risk factors, including dyslipidemia [55], increased blood pressure [56], arterial compliance [55], inflammation [57, 58] and vascular reactivity [59]. A recent meta-analysis showed that there were 9% and 13% risk reductions in coronary heart disease (CHD) events and myocardial infarction, respectively, with 1 g/day DHA supplements, and the effects were dose-dependent [60].

Earlier studies were done on the benefits of n- 3 LCPUFA in preventing CVD using a combination of EPA and DHA. In recent years, the separate effects of EPA and DHA on the risk factors of CVD have been shown in order to have a better understanding of their mechanisms. Asztalos et al. [60] recruited 121 healthy, normolipidemic subjects, where subjects were randomly assigned into four treatment groups: two doses of EPA (1800 and 600 mg/day), one dose of DHA (600 mg/day), and olive oil without EPA and DHA (control). After 6 weeks of intervention, the DHA group showed a significant decrease in the postprandial TG concentration compared with the control group although the fasting TG remained unchanged. However, interestingly, the DHA group also displays a significant increase in the low-density lipoprotein cholesterol (LDL) level. Although the EPA groups did not show the same results, there was a significant decrease in the lipoprotein-associated phospholipase A2 concentration, which is an inflammatory marker, at the dose of 1800 mg EPA/day. It seems that both EPA and DHA can decrease the CVD risk factors, and DHA may be more effective in reducing the lipid risk factors than EPA [61].

9. Cancers

Cancer is one of the most frequently diagnosed diseases worldwide, cancer is one of the leading causes of death in the Western world, and omega-3 fatty acids have long been claimed to reduce the risk of certain cancers. Interestingly, studies indicate that people who take the most omega-3s have up to a 55% lower risk of colon cancer [62, 63]. Additionally, omega-3 consumption is linked to a reduced risk of prostate cancer in men and breast cancer in women. However, not all studies show the same results [64–66].

10. Vision and eye health

Age-related macular degeneration is a major cause of blindness worldwide. With aging populations in many countries, more than 20% might have the disorder. DHA, a type of omega-3, is a key structural component of the retina of your eye [67]. When enough DHA is not present in the body, vision problems may arise [68, 69]. Interestingly having enough omega-3 is linked to a reduced risk of macular degeneration, one of the world's leading causes of permanent eye damage and blindness [69, 70].

11. Inflammatory bowel disease

The anti-inflammatory effects of omega-3 fats may assist in managing inflammatory bowel disease (IBD) and other gastrointestinal diseases causing inflammation, but the available evidence is weak [71, 72]. In one study, 4.2 g of fish oil daily for 8 months reduced the symptoms of active mild-to-moderate ulcerative colitis [73]. However, a review of three clinical trials and 138 ulcerative colitis patients found no significant benefits of fish oil supplementation. The authors suggested further trials with improved fish oil formulation (enteric-coated capsules) [74].

12. Depression and anxiety

Symptoms of depression include sadness, lethargy, and a general loss of interest in life [75]. Anxiety is also a common disorder and is characterized by constant worry and nervousness [76]. It is one of the most common mental disorders in the world. Interestingly, studies indicate that people who eat omega-3 s regularly are less likely to be depressed [77, 78]. What's more, when people with depression or anxiety start consuming omega-3 supplements, their symptoms improve [79, 80]. ALA, EPA, and DHA are the three types of omega-3 fatty acids. Of the three, EPA seems to be the best at fighting depression [81].

13. Improving ADHD

Attention deficit hyperactivity disorder (ADHD)—characterized by impulsive behaviors and difficulty concentrating—generally starts in childhood but often continues into adulthood [82]. As the main omega-3 fat in your brain, DHA helps boost blood flow during mental tasks. Research has demonstrated that children and adults with ADHD commonly have lower blood levels of DHA [82–84]. In a recent review, seven of nine studies that tested the effects of DHA supplements in children with ADHD give some improvement—such as with regard to attention or behavior [85]. For example, in a large 16-week study in 362 children, those taking 600 mg of DHA daily had an 8% decrease in impulsive behaviors as rated by their parents, which was twice the decrease observed in the placebo group [86]. In another 16-week study in 40 boys with ADHD, 650 mg each of DHA and EPA daily alongside the children's usual ADHD medication resulted in a 15% decrease in attention problems [87].

14. Metabolic syndrome

A metabolic syndrome is a group of conditions. It consists of central obesity—also known as belly fat—as well as high blood pressure, insulin resistance, high triglycerides, and low "good" HDL cholesterol levels. It is a major public health issue because it increases your risk of many other illnesses, including heart disease and diabetes [88]. Omega-3 fatty acids can help insulin resistance, inflammation, and heart disease risk factors in people with metabolic syndrome [80, 89, 90].

15. Skin health

DHA is a structural component of our skin. It is responsible for the health of cell membranes, which are up to a large part of your skin. A healthy cell membrane shows soft, moist, supple, and wrinkle-free skin. EPA also benefits the skin in several ways, including managing oil production, and skin hydration, and preventing hyperkeratinization of hair follicles, which appears as the little red bumps often seen on upper arms, reducing premature aging of your skin, reducing the risk of acne [91, 92]. Omega-3s can also save your skin from sun damage. EPA aids in blocking the release of substances that eat away at the collagen in your skin after sun exposure [91, 93].

16. Early preterm births

Delivering a baby before 34 weeks of pregnancy is known as early preterm birth and increases the baby's risk of health problems [94, 95]. An analysis of two large studies shows that women consuming 600–800 mg of DHA daily during pregnancy decreased their risk of early preterm birth by more than 40% in the US and 64% in Australia, compared to those taking a placebo [96]. Therefore, it is especially critical to make sure that you are getting sufficient amounts of DHA when you are pregnant—either through diet, supplements or both.

17. Age-related cognitive decline (ARCD) and Alzheimer's disease

Docosahexaenoic acid (DHA) has an important role in neural function. Decreases in plasma DHA are related to cognitive decline in healthy elderly adults and in patients with Alzheimer's disease. A higher DHA level is inversely correlated with a relative risk of Alzheimer's disease. Twenty-four-week supplementation with 900 mg/d DHA is reported to improve learning and memory function in ARCD and is a beneficial supplement that supports cognitive health with aging [97].

18. Kidney disorders

Researchers at the Mayo Clinic report that patients with IgA nephropathy have an abnormal EFA profile and that this abnormality can be corrected by supplementation with fish oil. The researchers conclude that fish oil supplementation retards the progression of IgA nephropathy [98]. Kidney transplant patients also benefit from fish oils [99].

19. Neuropathic pain

Pain is an electrical signal interpreted by one's brain. Neuropathic pain or nerve pain is a chronic pain state that usually (but not always) is caused by some sort of tissue trauma. In neuropathic pain, the nerve fibers themselves get often damaged, dysfunctional, or injured. These damaged nerve fibers transmit incorrect electrical signals to the brain's pain centers. The first-ever reported case series suggests that omega-3 fatty acids may be of benefit in the management of patients with neuropathic pain [100]. Long-chain omega-3 fatty acids supplementation accelerates nerve regeneration and prevents neuropathic pain behavior in mice [101]. Treatment with omega-3 PUFA could represent a promising therapeutic approach in the management of neurological injury [102].

20. Benefits for the aging brain

Brain volume shrinks with age [103], with a parallel decrease in DHA composition [104]. DHA is critical for healthy brain aging. With aging, your brain goes through natural changes, characterized by increased oxidative stress, altered energy metabolism, and DNA damage [105], while many of these changes are also seen when DHA levels decrease. These include altered membrane properties, enzyme activity, memory function, and neuron function [106]. Importantly, n-3 PUFA intake is positively correlated with gray matter volume in adults [107] and in brain regions responsible for cognition in normal, elderly adults [108]. Taking a supplement may help, as DHA supplements have been linked to significant improvements in memory, learning, and verbal fluency in those with mild memory complaints [108]. Environmental factors, such as diet, exercise, and DHA consumption, can positively affect the normal aging process and overall mental health and performance [109].

21. Benefits of asthma in children

Asthma is a chronic lung disease, which has symptoms like coughing, shortness of breath, and wheezing. Severe asthma attacks can have very dangerous attacks. They are characterized by inflammation and swelling in the airways of your lungs. Specialized pro-resolving mediators (SPM: protectins, resolvins, and maresins) are released from omega-3 fatty acids, such as EPA and DHA, *via* several enzymatic reactions. These mediators counter-regulate airway eosinophilic inflammation and promote the resolution of inflammation *in vivo* [110, 111]. Several studies link omega-3 consumption with a lower risk of asthma in children and young adults [112, 113].

22. Fat reduction in liver

Nonalcoholic fatty liver disease (NAFLD) is more common than you think. It has increased with the obesity epidemic to become the most common cause of chronic liver disease in the Western world [114]. However, supplementing with omega-3 fatty acids effectively decreases liver fat and inflammation in people with NAFLD [115].

23. Psychosis

In a study of 81 young patients with mild psychosis, low-dose omega-3 supplementation (1.2 g/day) significantly reduced the incidence of psychotic disorders [94]. Further trials should investigate this potential benefit of omega-3/fish oil.

24. Cachexia

Taking mega-doses (7.5–8.1 g daily) of fish oil slightly slowed down weight loss in 67 patients with cancer-related cachexia (severe weakness and wasting) [116, 117]. Lower doses (3 g daily) do not seem to have beneficial effects [118].

25. Aggression

DHA significantly reduced aggression due to mental stress in a study of 41 students. The same group of authors failed to confirm this benefit in non-stressful situations [119, 120]. In a 6-month study on 200 school children aged 8–16 years old, omega-3 supplementation caused a significant reduction in several measures of aggression [121].

26. Rheumatoid arthritis

Resolvins found in EPA and DHA appear to prevent certain inflammatory cytokines, such as TNF-α from inducing pain [122]. Long-term supplementation with fish oils benefits rheumatoid arthritis patients significantly and may lessen their need for NSAIDs and other RA medications [123]. Dietary fish oil supplements should now be regarded as part of standard therapy for rheumatoid arthritis [124, 125].

27. Osteoporosis and bone health

Osteoporosis and arthritis are two common disorders that affect your skeletal system. Studies show that omega-3 s can improve bone strength by boosting the amount of calcium in your bones, which should lead to a reduced risk of osteoporosis [126, 127]. Omega-3 s may also cure arthritis. Patients taking omega-3 supplements have been reported to have reduced joint pain and increased grip strength [128, 129].

28. Omega-3s and menstrual pain

Menstrual pain occurs in your lower abdomen and pelvis and often radiates to your lower back and thighs. It can significantly affect the quality of female life. However, studies repeatedly prove that women who consume the most omega-3s have milder menstrual pain [129, 130]. One study even determined that an omega-3 supplement was more effective than ibuprofen in treating severe pain during menstruation [131].

29. Good sleep

Good sleep is one foundation for good health. Low levels of omega-3 fatty acids are associated with sleep problems in children and obstructive sleep apnea in adults [131, 132]. Low levels of DHA are also linked to lower levels of the hormone melatonin, which helps you fall asleep [133]. Studies in both children and adults reveal that supplementing with omega-3 increases the length and quality of sleep [132, 133].

30. Blood pressure reduction and circulation help

DHA boosts good blood flow, or circulation, and may help endothelial function—the ability of your blood vessels to dilate [134]. A review of 20 studies found that DHA and EPA may also help in lowering blood pressure, though each specific fat may affect different aspects. DHA decreases diastolic blood pressure (the bottom number of a reading) by an average of 3.1 mmHg, while EPA helps lower systolic blood pressure (the top number of a reading) by an average of 3.8 mmHg [135].

31. DHA in sport nutrition

DHA may influence sports performance by improving aerobic processes and using fat as an energy substrate [136]. The applications of omega-3 supplementation for sports performance seem to be relevant for athletes involved in strength, endurance, and team-based activities. However, determining exactly how they work and how much omega-3s may benefit strength, endurance, and recovery is not confirmed. This is accomplished by enhancing the delivery of oxygen and nutrients and removing waste products from tissues. Postexercise recovery time may decrease due to reduced inflammation and increased release of growth hormones [137].

Walser et al. [137], reported that stroke volume and cardiac output increased during exercise when DHA + EPA were administered to subjects. This finding suggests that DHA + EPA may increase oxygen delivery during exercise [138]. Other researchers have shown that DHA + EPA supplementation improves circulatory function through. DHA supplementation improves minute heart rate recovery after exercise. Both of these DHA-related effects may contribute to better athletic performance and exercise recovery. DHA supplementation during exercise positively affects cognition and the strength of the connection between synapses in the brain [139].

32. DHA and skeletal muscle

Skeletal muscle disuse results in a reduction in fed and fasted rates of skeletal muscle protein synthesis, leading to the loss of skeletal muscle mass. Recent evidence has shown that supplementation with ω-3 fatty acids during a period of skeletal muscle disuse increases the ω-3 fatty acid composition of skeletal muscle membranes, heightens rates of skeletal muscle protein synthesis, and protects against skeletal muscle loss. Omega-3 fatty acid ingestion is a potential preventive therapy to combat skeletal muscle-disuse atrophy but additional, appropriately powered randomized controlled trials are now needed in a range of populations before firm conclusions can be made [140]. Following n3-PUFA supplementation, mixed muscle, mitochondrial, and sarcoplasmic protein synthesis rates were moved up higher in older adults before exercise. n3-PUFA boosts postexercise mitochondrial and myofibrillar protein synthesis in older adults. These results have shown that n3-PUFA reduces mitochondrial oxidant emissions, increases postabsorptive muscle protein synthesis, and enhances anabolic responses to exercise in older adults [141]. Enrichment of EPA and DHA in these membrane phospholipids is linked to enhanced rates of muscle protein synthesis, decreased expression of factors that regulate muscle protein breakdown, and improved mitochondrial respiration kinetics [141].

33. Men's reproductive and sexual health

As wellness professionals would agree, fish oil does help with sexual performance and more. They would recommend filling up with the omega-3 in fish oil every day to be empowered sexually with maximum energy and drive. Neurons, photoreceptor cells, and spermatozoa are three cell types that show high DHA content. The structural integrity of the spermatozoa cell membrane plays a pivotal role in successful fertilization. This is because both the acrosome reaction and sperm-oocyte fusion is associated with the membrane's fatty acid profile [142].

The majority of researchers have demonstrated that DHA (22:6n-3) is a major PUFA in human spermatozoa. Its deficiency is a typical sign in spermatozoa of subfertile or infertile men [143]. DHA comprises up to 30% of esterified fatty acids in phospholipids and 73% of all PUFAs and it gives proper fluidity to fertile sperm [142]. The percentage of DHA in sperm membrane phospholipids was higher than that of DHA in other cells. Hence, PUFA metabolism was more active in the testes during spermatogenesis and epididymal sperm maturation than these PUFA metabolism in other cells [144]. Interestingly, Zalata et al. have indicated that DHA in human spermatozoa may have specific functions unrelated to fluidity, which is similar to the functions of DHA in the brain and retina. More recently, it has been suggested that lipid concentrations may affect semen parameters, and this effect is more pronounced in sperm head morphology [145] Inadequate DHA concentration is the main cause of low-quality spermatozoa. Getting adequate DHA supports both the vitality and motility of sperm and improves sperm quality and function, which impacts fertility [142].

For erectile dysfunction, consuming a fish oil concentrate improves blood flow to the pelvis, reduces inflammation, and cuts the risk of tiny blood clots that impede erections. Highly absorbable omega-3 fats in a concentrate also stabilize hormone and neurotransmitter balance, for stronger erections that are sustained longer [146]. A healthy heart is a good sign of a functioning penis.

"Many of our male patients over the years are receiving enduring improvements in erectile dysfunction, taking a potent fish oil concentrate for at least 6 months."—Dr. Rachelle Herdman.

34. Benefits for healthy hair growth

Fatty acids promote hair growth, as well as add sheen and luster to hair. A proper amount of omega-3 in your diet prevents dry, itchy, flaky scalp, and is beneficial in reversing hair loss [147].

35. Help in stem cells

Omega-3 fatty acids support stem cells [148]. The available evidence shows that n-6 and n-3 PUFA and their metabolites can act through multiple mechanisms to promote the proliferation and differentiation of various stem cell types [149].

36. Conclusion

In summary, the health benefits of DHA start from the baby's formation in the mother's womb and continue to the adolescent and adult stages up to aging for men and women, including sexual health. Higher DHA levels in body are associated with better mental, physical health, and performance enhancement while low level of DHA has been linked to physical and mental diseases that may cost huge financial burdens. So, DHA is a critical component for a happy life. There have been negative results in a few human trials of the effectiveness of omega-3 fatty acids starting from even CVD. However, the substantial literature of positive results outweighs the negative results. It will be wiser for us to keep the optimum level of DHA in our bodies throughout life. Indeed, it needs more research to verify them more.

Acknowledgements

Authors acknowledge gratefully the initiation of IntechOpen .com team for the book and the typist for his help.

Author details

Abdul Hei* and Laishram Sanahanbi
Lilong Haoreibi College, Lilong, Manipur, India

*Address all correspondence to: ahei541@gmail.com

References

[1] Shahidi F, Ambigaipalan P. Omega-3 polyunsaturated fatty acids and their health benefits. Annual Review of Food Science and Technology. 2018;**9**:345-381. DOI: 10.1146/annurev-food-111317-095850

[2] Hashimoto M, Hossain S, Al Mamun A, Matsuzaki K, Arai H. Docosahexaenoic acid: One molecule diverse functions. Critical Reviews in Biotechnology. 2017;**37**(5):579-597. DOI: 10.1080/07388551.2016.1207153

[3] Bradbury J. Docosahexaenoic acid (DHA): An ancient nutrient for the modern human brain. Nutrients. 2011;**3**(5):529-554. DOI: 10.3390/nu3050529. Epub 2011 May 10

[4] Swanson D, Block R, Mousa SA. Omega-3 fatty acids EPA and DHA: Health benefits throughout life. Advances in Nutrition. 2012;**3**(1):1-7. DOI: 10.3945/an.111.000893. Epub 2012 Jan 5

[5] Frits A. J. Muskiet, M. Rebecca Fokkema, Anne Schaafsma, E. Rudy Boersma and Michael A. Crawford Issues and Opinion, Is Docosahexaenoic Acid (DHA) Essential? Lessons from DHA Status Regulation, Our Ancient Diet, Epidemiology and andomized Controlled trials. Available from: https:/academic.uop.com/jn/article/134/1/183/4688233 [Accessed: February 05, 2020]

[6] Nutrition, DHA (Docosahexaenoic Acid): A Detailed Review. Available from: https://www.healthline.com/nutrition/dha-docosahexaenoic-acid#what-it-is [Accessed: September 15, 2022]

[7] Sarojnalini C, Hei A. Fish as an important functional food for quality life. In: Lagouri V, editor. Functional Foods. London: IntechOpen; 2019. DOI: 10.5772/intechopen.81947

[8] Weiser MJ, Butt CM, Mohajeri MH. Docosahexaenoic acid and cognition throughout the lifespan. Nutrients. 2016;**8**(2):99. DOI: 10.3390/nu8020099

[9] Igarashi M, Ma K, Chang L, Bell JM, Rapoport SI. Rat heart cannot synthesize docosahexaenoic acid from circulating alpha-linolenic acid because it lacks elongase-2. Journal of Lipid Research. 2008;**49**:1735-1745. DOI: 10.1194/jlr.M800093-JLR200

[10] Rodriguez-Leyva D, Bassett CM, McCullough R, Pierce GN. The cardiovascular effects of flaxseed and its omega-3 fatty acid, alpha-linolenic acid. Canadian Journal of Cardiology. 2010;**26**(9):489-496. DOI: 10.1016/S0828-282X(10)70455-4

[11] Watters CA, Edmonds CM, Rosner LS, Sloss KP, Leung P. A cost analysis of EPA and DHA in fish, supplements and foods. Journal of Nutrition & Food Sciences. 2012;**2**(8):159. DOI: 10.4172/2155-9600.1000159

[12] Inhamuns AJ, Franco MRB. EPA and DHA quantification in two species of freshwater fish from central Amazonia. Food Chemistry. 2008;**107**(2):587-591. DOI: 10.1016/j.foodchem.2007.07.032

[13] Echeverría F, Valenzuela R, Hernandez-Rodas MC, Valenzuela A. Docosahexaenoic acid (DHA), a fundamental fatty acid for the brain: New dietary sources. Prostaglandins, Leukotrienes, and Essential Fatty Acids. 2017;**124**:1-10. DOI: 10.1016/j.plefa.2017.08.001

[14] Garg P, Pejaver RK, Sukhija M, Ahuja A. Role of DHA, ARA, & phospholipids in brain development: An Indian perspective. Clinical Epidemiology and Global Health. 2017;**5**(4):155-162. ISSN 2213-3984

[15] Li J, Pora BLR, Dong K, Hasjim J. Health benefits of docosahexaenoic acid and its bioavailability: A review. Food Science & Nutrition. 2021;**9**(9):5229-5243. DOI: 10.1002/fsn3.2299

[16] Horrocks LA, Yeo YK. Health benefits of docosahexaenoic acid (DHA). Pharmacological Research. 1999;**40**(3):211-225. DOI: 10.1006/phrs.1999.0495

[17] Shahidi F, Ambigaipalan P. Novel functional food ingredients from marine sources. Current Opinion in Food Science. 2015;**2**:123-129

[18] Shahidi F, Ambigaipalan P. Beverages fortified with omega 3 fatty acids, dietary fiber, minerals and vitamins. In: Shahidi F, Alsalvar C, editors. Handbook of Functional Beverages and Human Health. Boca Raton, FL: CRC Pres; 2016. pp. 801-813

[19] Finley JW, Shahidi F. The chemistry, processing, and health benefits of highly unsaturated fatty acids:an overview. In: Shahidi F, Finely JW, editors. Omega-3 Fatty Acids. Washington, DC: ACS; 2001. pp. 2-11

[20] Lopez LB, Kritz-Silverstein D, Barrett-Connor E. High dietary and plasma levels of the omega-3 fatty acid docosahexaenoic acid are associated with decreased dementia risk: The Rancho Bernardo study. Journal of Nutrition, Health and Aging. 2011;**15**:25-31

[21] Calder PC. Docosahexaenoic acid. Annals of Nutrition & Metabolism. 2016;**69**(Suppl 1):7-21. DOI: 10.1159/000448262. Epub 2016 Nov 15

[22] Basak S, Mallick R, Duttaroy AK. Maternal docosahexaenoic acid status during pregnancy and its impact on infant neurodevelopment. Nutrients. 2020;**12**(12):3615. DOI: 10.3390/nu12123615

[23] Lauritzen L, Hansen HS, Jørgensen MH, Michaelsen KF. The essentiality of long chain n-3 fatty acids in relation to development and function of the brain and retina. Progress in Lipid Research. 2001;**40**:1-94

[24] Valentine CJ. Maternal dietary DHA supplementation to improve inflammatory outcomes in the preterm infant. Advances in Nutrition. 2012;**3**:370-376

[25] Tosi F, Sartori F, Guarini P, Olivieri O, Martinelli N. Delta-5 and delta-6 desaturases: Crucial enzymes in polyunsaturated fatty acid-related pathways with pleiotropic influences in health and disease. Advances in Experimental Medicine and Biology. 2014;**824**:61-81

[26] Khalida W, Gillb P, Arshada MS, Alic A, Muhammad, Ranjhad MAN, et al. Functional behavior of DHA and EPA in the formation of babies brain at different stages of age, and protect from different brain-related diseases. International Journal of Food Properties. 2022;**25**(1):1021-1044. DOI: 10.1080/10942912.2022.2070642

[27] Helland IB, Smith L, Blomen B, Saarem K, Saugstad OD, Drevon CA. Effect of supplementing pregnant and lactating mothers with n-3 very- long-chain fatty acids on children's IQ and body mass index at 7 years of age. Pediatrics. 2008;**122**:e472-e479

[28] Dunstan JA, Simmer K, Dixon G, Prescott SL. Cognitive assessment of children at age 2(1/2) years after maternal fish oil supplementation in pregnancy: A randomised controlled trial. Archives of Disease in Childhood. Fetal and Neonatal Edition. 2008;**93**:F45-F50

[29] Judge MP, Harel O, Lammi-Keefe CJ. Maternal consumption of a docosahexaenoic acid-containing functional food during pregnancy: Benefit for infant performance on problem-solving but not on recognition memory tasks at age 9 mo. The American Journal of Clinical Nutrition. 2007;**85**:1572-1577

[30] Leaf DA, Hatcher L. The effect of lean fish consumption on triglyceride levels. The Physician and Sportsmedicine. 2009;**37**:37-43

[31] Hadley KB, Ryan AS, Forsyth S, Gautier S, Salem N. The essentiality of arachidonic acid in infant development. Nutrients. 2016;**8**:216

[32] Lauritzen L, Brambilla P, Mazzocchi A, Harsløf LB, Ciappolino V, Agostoni C. DHA effects in brain development and function. Nutrients. 2016;**8**(1):6. DOI: 10.3390/nu8010006

[33] Lauritzen L, Jorgensen MH, Olsen SF, Straarup EM, Michaelsen KF. Maternal fish oil supplementation in lactation: Effect on developmental outcome in breast-fed infants. Reproduction, Nutrition, Development. 2005;**45**(5):535-547

[34] Willatts P, Forsyth JS, DiModugno MK, Varma S, Colvin M. Effect of long-chain polyunsaturated fatty acids in infant formula on problem solving at 10 months of age. Lancet. 1998;**352**(9129):688-691

[35] Gustafsson PA, Duchen K, Birberg U, Karlsson T. Breastfeeding, very long polyunsaturated fatty acids (PUFA) and IQ at 6 1/2 years of age. Acta Paediatrica. 2004;**93**(10):1280-1287

[36] Auestad N, Scott DT, Janowsky JS, et al. Visual, cognitive, and language assessments at 39 months: A follow-up study of children fed formulas containing long-chain polyunsaturated fatty acids to 1 year of age. Pediatrics. 2003;**112**(3 Pt 1):e177-e183

[37] Innis SM. Polyunsaturated fatty acids in human milk: An essential role in infant development. Advances in Experimental Medicine and Biology. 2004;**554**:27-43

[38] Lauritzen L, Jorgensen MH, Mikkelsen TB, et al. Maternal fish oil supplementation in lactation: Effect on visual acuity and n-3 fatty acid content of infant erythrocytes. Lipids. 2004;**39**(3):195-206

[39] Helland IB, Saugstad OD, Smith L, et al. Similar effects on infants of n-3 and n-6 fatty acids supplementation to pregnant and lactating women. Pediatrics. 2001;**108**(5):E82

[40] Lauritzen L, Hoppe C, Straarup EM, Michaelsen KF. Maternal fish oil supplementation in lactation and growth during the first 2.5 years of life. Pediatric Research. 2005;**58**(2):235-242

[41] Carlson SE, Colombo J, Gajewski BJ, Gustafson KM, Mundy D, Yeast J, et al. DHA supplementation and pregnancy outcomes. The American Journal of Clinical Nutrition. 2013;**97**(4):808-815. DOI: 10.3945/ajcn.112.050021. Epub 2013 Feb 20

[42] Rogers LK, Valentine CJ, Keim SA. DHA supplementation: Current implications in pregnancy and childhood. Pharmacological Research.

2013;**70**(1):13-19. DOI: 10.1016/j.phrs.2012.12.003. Epub 2012 Dec 21

[43] Calder PC. Omega-3 fatty acids and inflammatory processes. Nutrients. 2010;**2**(3):355-374. DOI: 10.3390/nu2030355. Epub 2010 Mar 18

[44] Calder PC. Fatty acids and inflammation: The cutting edge between food and pharma. European Journal of Pharmacology. 2011;**668**(Suppl 1):S50-S58. DOI: 10.1016/j.ejphar.2011.05.085. Epub 2011 Jul 28

[45] Calder PC. Long-chain fatty acids and inflammation. The Proceedings of the Nutrition Society. 2012;**71**(2):284-289. DOI: 10.1017/S0029665112000067. Epub 2012 Feb 28

[46] Calder PC. Omega-3 fatty acids and inflammatory processes: From molecules to man. Biochemical Society Transactions. 2017;**45**(5):1105-1115. DOI: 10.1042/BST20160474. Epub 2017 Sep 12

[47] Fritsche KL. The science of fatty acids and inflammation. Advances in Nutrition. 2015;**6**(3):293S-301S. DOI: 10.3945/an.114.006940

[48] Lee JY, Zhao L, Hwang DH. Modulation of pattern recognition receptor-mediated inflammation and risk of chronic diseases by dietary fatty acids. Nutrition Reviews. 2010;**68**:38-61

[49] Sreeniwas Kumar A, Sinha N. Cardiovascular disease in India: A 60 degree overview. Medical Journal, Armed Forces India. 2020;**76**(1):1-3. DOI: 10.1016/j.mjafi.2019.12.005. Epub 2020 Jan 13

[50] American Heart Association. CVD Report. Available from: https://www.heart.org/en/get-involved/advocate/federal-priorities/cardiovascular-disease-burden-report [Accessed: September 16, 2022]

[51] Mozaffarian D, JHY W. Omega-3 fatty acids and cardio-vascular disease: Effects on risk factors, molecular pathways, and clinical events. Journal of the American College of Cardiology. 2011;**58**(20):2047-2067

[52] Schmidt EB, Arnesen H, De Caterina R, Rasmussen LH, Kristensen SD. Marine *n*-3 polyunsaturated fatty acids and coronary heart disease: Part I. Background, epidemiology, animal data, effects on risk factors and safety. Thrombosis Research. 2005;**115**(3):163-170

[53] Dawczynski C, Martin L, Wagner A, Jahreis G. *N*-3 LC-PUFA enriched dairy products are able to reduce cardiovascular risk factors: A double-blind, cross-over study. Clinical Nutrition. 2010;**29**(5):592-599. DOI: 10.1016/j.clnu.2010.02.008

[54] Nestel P, Shige H, Pomeroy S, Cehun M, Abbey M, Raederstorff D. The *n*-3 fatty acids eicosapentaenoic acid and docosahexaenoic acid increase systemic arterial compliance in humans. American Journal of Clinical Nutrition. 2002;**76**(2):326-330

[55] Geleijnse JM, Giltay EJ, Grobbee DE, Donders ART, Kok FJ. Blood pressure response to fish oil supplementation: Metaregression analysis of randomized trials. Journal of Hypertension. 2002;**20**(8):1493-1499. DOI: 10.1097/00004872-200208000-00010

[56] Ebrahimi M, Ghayour-Mobarhan M, Rezaiean S, Hoseini M, Parizade SMR, Farhoudi F, et al. Omega-3 fatty acid supplements improve the cardiovascular risk profile of subjects with metabolic syndrome, including markers of

inflammation and auto-immunity. Acta Cardiologica. 2009;**64**(3):321-327

[57] Mori TA, Burke V, Puddey IB, Watts GF, O'Neal DN, Best JD, et al. Purified eicosapentaenoic and docosahexae-noic acids have differential effects on serum lipids and lipoproteins, LDL particle size, glucose, and insulin in mildly hyperlipidemic men. The American Journal of Clinical Nutrition. 2000;**71**(5):1085-1094. DOI: 10.1016/S0021-9150(00)80500-6

[58] Mori TA, Watts GF, Burke V, Hilme E, Puddey IB, Beilin LJ. Differential effects of eicosapentaenoic acid and docosahexaenoic acid on vascular reactivity of the forearm microcirculation in hyperlipidemic, overweight men. Circulation. 2000;**102**(11):1264-1269

[59] Bernasconi AA, Wiest MM, Lavie CJ, Milani RV, Laukkanen JA. Effect of Omega-3 dosage on cardiovascular outcomes: An updated meta-analysis and meta-regression of interventional trials. Mayo Clinic Proceedings. 2001;**96**(2):304-313

[60] Asztalos IB, Gleason JA, Sever S, Gedik R, Asztalos BF, Horvath KV, et al. Effects of eicosapentaenoic acid and docosahexaenoic acid on cardiovascular disease risk factors: A randomized clinical trial. Metabolism. 2016;**65**(11):1636-1645

[61] Theodoratou E, McNeill G, Cetnarskyj R, Farrington SM, Tenesa A, Barnetson R, et al. Dietary fatty acids and colorectal cancer: A case-control study. American Journal of Epidemiology. 2007;**166**(2):181-195. DOI: 10.1093/aje/kwm063. Epub 2007 May 9

[62] Zhong X, Fang YJ, Pan ZZ, Li B, Wang L, Zheng MC, et al. Dietary fat, fatty acid intakes and colorectal cancer risk in Chinese adults: A case-control study. European Journal of Cancer Prevention. 2013;**22**(5):438-447. DOI: 10.1097/CEJ.0b013e32835e88c4

[63] Terry PD, Terry JB, Rohan TE. Long-chain (n-3) fatty acid intake and risk of cancers of the breast and the prostate: Recent epidemiological studies, biological mechanisms, and directions for future research. The Journal of Nutrition. 2004;**134**(12 Suppl):3412S-3420S. DOI: 10.1093/jn/134.12.3412S

[64] Fabian CJ, Kimler BF, Hursting SD. Omega-3 fatty acids for breast cancer prevention and survivorship. Breast Cancer Research. 2015;**17**(1):62. DOI: 10.1186/s13058-015-0571-6

[65] Kaizer L, Boyd NF, Kriukov V, Tritchler D. Fish consumption and breast cancer risk: An ecological study. Nutrition and Cancer. 1989;**12**(1):61-68. DOI: 10.1080/01635588909514002

[66] Anderson GJ, Connor WE, Corliss JD. Docosahexaenoic acid is the preferred dietary n-3 fatty acid for the development of the brain and retina. Pediatric Research. 1990;**27**(1):89-97. DOI: 10.1203/00006450-199001000-00023

[67] Singh M. Essential fatty acids, DHA and human brain. Indian Journal of Pediatrics. 2005;**72**(3):239-242

[68] SanGiovanni JP, Chew EY. The role of omega-3 long-chain polyunsaturated fatty acids in health and disease of the retina. Progress in Retinal and Eye Research. 2005;**24**(1):87-138. DOI: 10.1016/j.preteyeres.2004.06.002

[69] Merle BM, Benlian P, Puche N, Bassols A, Delcourt C, Souied EH, et al. Circulating omega-3 fatty acids and neovascular age-related macular degeneration. Investigative Ophthalmology & Visual Science.

2014;**55**(3):2010-2019. DOI: 10.1167/iovs.14-13916

[70] Lim LS, Mitchell P, Seddon JM, Holz FG, Wong TY. Age-related macular degeneration. Lancet. 2012;**379**(9827):1728-1738. DOI: 10.1016/S0140-6736(12)60282-7

[71] Farrukh A, Mayberry JF. Is there a role for managing inflammatory bowel disease (IBD) and other gastrointestinal diseases causing inflammation, but the available evidence fish oil in inflammatory bowel disease? World Journal of Clinical Cases. 2014;**2**(7):250-252. DOI: 10.12998/wjcc.v2.i7.250

[72] Aslan A, Triadafilopoulos G. Fish oil fatty acid supplementation in active ulcerative colitis: A double-blind, placebo-controlled, crossover study. The American Journal of Gastroenterology. 1992;**87**(4):432-437

[73] Turner D, Steinhart AH, Griffiths AM. Omega 3 fatty acids (fish oil) for maintenance of remission in ulcerative colitis. Cochrane Database of Systematic Reviews. 2007;(3):CD006443. DOI: 10.1002/14651858.CD006443.pub2

[74] Wani AL, Bhat SA, Ara A. Omega-3 fatty acids and the treatment of depression: A review of scientific evidence. Integrative Medicine Research. 2015;**4**(3):132-141. ISSN 2213-4220

[75] Kessler RC, Chiu WT, Demler O, Merikangas KR, Walters EE. Prevalence, severity, and comorbidity of 12-month DSM-IV disorders in the National Comorbidity Survey Replication. Archives of General Psychiatry. 2005;**62**(6):617-627. DOI: 10.1001/archpsyc.62.6.617. Erratum in: Archives of General Psychiatry 2005;62(7):709. Merikangas, Kathleen R [added]

[76] Grosso G, Galvano F, Marventano S, Malaguarnera M, Bucolo C, Drago F, et al. Omega-3 fatty acids and depression: Scientific evidence and biological mechanisms. Oxidative Medicine and Cellular Longevity. 2014;**2014**:313570. DOI: 10.1155/2014/313570. Epub 2014 Mar 18

[77] Lin PY, Su KP. A meta-analytic review of double-blind, placebo-controlled trials of antidepressant efficacy of omega-3 fatty acids. The Journal of Clinical Psychiatry. 2007;**68**(7):1056-1061. DOI: 10.4088/jcp.v68n0712

[78] Ginty AT, Conklin SM. Short-term supplementation of acute long-chain omega-3 polyunsaturated fatty acids may alter depression status and decrease symptomology among young adults with depression: A preliminary randomized and placebo controlled trial. Psychiatry Research. 2015;**229**(1-2):485-489. ISSN 0165-1781

[79] Su K-P, Huang S-Y, Chiu C-C, Shen WW. Omega-3 fatty acids in major depressive disorder: A preliminary double-blind, placebo-controlled trial. European Neuropsychopharmacology. 2003;**13**(4):267-271

[80] Kiecolt-Glaser JK, Belury MA, Andridge R, Malarkey WB, Glaser R. Omega-3 supplementation lowers inflammation and anxiety in medical students: A randomized controlled trial. Brain, Behavior, and Immunity. 2011;**25**(8):1725-1734. DOI: 10.1016/j.bbi.2011.07.229. Epub 2011 Jul 19

[81] Mozaffari-Khosravi H, Yassini-Ardakani M, Karamati M, Shariati-Bafghi SE. Eicosapentaenoic acid versus docosahexaenoic acid in mild-to-moderate depression: A randomized, double-blind, placebo-controlled trial.

European Neuropsychopharmacology. 2013;**23**(7):636-644. DOI: 10.1016/j.euroneuro.2012.08.003

[82] Bonvicini C, Faraone SV, Scassellati C. Attention-deficit hyperactivity disorder in adults: A systematic review and meta-analysis of genetic, pharmacogenetic and biochemical studies. Molecular Psychiatry. 2016;**21**(7):872-884. DOI: 10.1038/mp.2016.74. Epub 2016 May 24. Erratum in: Molecular Psychiatry. 2016;**21**(11):1643

[83] Königs A, Kiliaan AJ. Critical appraisal of omega-3 fatty acids in attention-deficit/hyperactivity disorder treatment. Neuropsychiatric Disease and Treatment. 2016;**12**:1869-1882. DOI: 10.2147/NDT.S68652

[84] Chen JR, Hsu SF, Hsu CD, Hwang LH, Yang SC. Dietary patterns and blood fatty acid composition in children with attention-deficit hyperactivity disorder in Taiwan. The Journal of Nutritional Biochemistry. 2004;**15**(8):467-472. DOI: 10.1016/j.jnutbio.2004.01.008

[85] Ramalho R, Pereira AC, Vicente F, Pereira P. Docosahexaenoic acid supplementation for children with attention deficit hyperactivity disorder: A comprehensive review of the evidence. Clinical Nutrition ESPEN. 2018;**25**:1-7. DOI: 10.1016/j.clnesp.2018.03.126

[86] Richardson AJ, Burton JR, Sewell RP, Spreckelsen TF, Montgomery P. Docosahexaenoic acid for reading, cognition and behavior in children aged 7-9 years: A randomized, controlled trial (the DOLAB Study). PLoS One. 2012;7(9):e43909. DOI: 10.1371/journal.pone.0043909. Epub 2012 Sep 6

[87] Bos DJ, Oranje B, Veerhoek ES, Van Diepen RM, Weusten JM, Demmelmair H, et al. Reduced symptoms of inattention after dietary omega-3 fatty acid supplementation in boys with and without attention deficit/hyperactivity disorder. Neuropsychopharmacology. 2015;**40**(10):2298-2306. DOI: 10.1038/npp.2015.73

[88] Kaur J. A comprehensive review on metabolic syndrome. Cardiology Research and Practice. 2014;**2014**:943162. DOI: 10.1155/2014/943162. Epub 2014 Mar 11. Retraction in: Cardiology Research and Practice. 2019;**2019**:4301528

[89] Robinson LE, Mazurak VC. N-3 polyunsaturated fatty acids: Relationship to inflammation in healthy adults and adults exhibiting features of metabolic syndrome. Lipids. 2013;**48**(4):319-332. DOI: 10.1007/s11745-013-3774-6. Epub 2013 Mar 1

[90] Dangardt F, Osika W, Chen Y, Nilsson U, Gan LM, Gronowitz E, et al. Omega-3 fatty acid supplementation improves vascular function and reduces inflammation in obese adolescents. Atherosclerosis. 2010;**212**(2):580-585. DOI: 10.1016/j.atherosclerosis.2010.06.046. Epub 2010 Jul 21

[91] Spencer EH, Ferdowsian HR, Barnard ND. Diet and acne: A review of the evidence. International Journal of Dermatology. 2009;**48**(4):339-347. DOI: 10.1111/j.1365-4632.2009.04002.x

[92] McCusker MM, Jane M. Grant-Kels Healing fats of the skin: The structural and immunologic roles of the ω-6 and ω-3 fatty acids. Clinics in Dermatology. 2010;**28**(4):440-451

[93] Fischer MA, Black HS. Modification of membrane composition, eicosanoid metabolism, and

immunoresponsiveness by dietary omega-3 and omega-6 fatty acid sources, modulators of ultraviolet-carcinogenesis. Photochemistry and Photobiology. 1991;**54**(3):381-387. DOI: 10.1111/j.1751-1097.1991.tb02031.x

[94] Amminger GP, Schäfer MR, Papageorgiou K, Klier CM, Cotton SM, Harrigan SM, et al. Long-chain omega-3 fatty acids for indicated prevention of psychotic disorders: A randomized, placebo-controlled trial. Archives of General Psychiatry. 2010;**67**(2):146-154. DOI: 10.1001/archgenpsychiatry.2009.192

[95] Shireman TI, Kerling EH, Gajewski BJ, Colombo J, Carlson SE. Docosahexaenoic acid supplementation (DHA) and the return on investment for pregnancy outcomes. Prostaglandins, Leukotrienes, and Essential Fatty Acids. 2016;**111**:8-10. DOI: 10.1016/j.plefa.2016.05.008

[96] Yelland LN, Gajewski BJ, Colombo J, Gibson RA, Makrides M, Carlson SE. Predicting the effect of maternal docosahexaenoic acid (DHA) supplementation to reduce early preterm birth in Australia and the United States using results of within country randomized controlled trials. Prostaglandins, Leukotrienes, and Essential Fatty Acids. 2016;**112**:44-49. DOI: 10.1016/j.plefa.2016.08.007

[97] Docosahexaenoic acid (DHA) plays an important role in neural function. Decreases in plasma DHA are associated with cognitive decline in healthy elderly adults and in patients with Alzheimer's disease. Higher DHA intake is inversely correlated with relative risk of Alzheimer's disease. The potential benefits of DHA supplementation in age-related cognitive decline (ARCD) have not been fully examined.

[98] Holman RT et al. Essential fatty acid deficiency profiles in idiopathic immunoglobulin A nephropathy. American Journal of Kidney Diseases. May 1994;**24**:648-654

[99] Ng R. Fish oil therapy in recurrent IgA nephropathy. Annals of Internal Medicine. 2003;**138**:1011-1012

[100] Ko GD, Nowacki NB, Arseneau L, Eitel M, Hum A. Omega-3 fatty acids for neuropathic pain: Case series. The Clinical Journal of Pain. 2010;**26**(2):168-172. DOI: 10.1097/AJP.0b013e3181bb8533

[101] Michael-Titus AT. Omega-3 fatty acids and neurological injury. Prostaglandins, Leukotrienes, and Essential Fatty Acids. 2007;**77**(5-6):295-300. DOI: 10.1016/j.plefa.2007.10.021

[102] Silva RV, Oliveira JT, Santos BLR, Dias FC, Martinez AMB, Lima CKF, et al. Long-chain omega-3 fatty acids supplementation accelerates nerve regeneration and prevents neuropathic pain behavior in mice. Frontiers in Pharmacology. 2017;**8**:723. DOI: 10.3389/fphar.2017.00723

[103] Resnick SM, Pham DL, Kraut MA, Zonderman AB, Davatzikos C. Longitudinal magnetic resonance imaging studies of older adults: A shrinking brain. The Journal of Neuroscience. 2003;**23**:3295-3301

[104] McNamara RK, Liu Y, Jandacek R, Rider T, Tso P. The aging human orbitofrontal cortex: Decreasing polyunsaturated fatty acid composition and associated increases in lipogenic gene expression and stearoyl-CoA desaturase activity. Prostaglandins, Leukotrienes and Essential Fatty Acids. 2008;**78**:293-304. DOI: 10.1016/j.plefa.2008.04.001

[105] Salem N Jr, Vandal M, Calon F. The benefit of docosahexaenoic acid for

the adult brain in aging and dementia. Prostaglandins, Leukotrienes, and Essential Fatty Acids. 2015;**92**:15-22. DOI: 10.1016/j.plefa.2014.10.003

[106] Canugovi C, Misiak M, Ferrarelli LK, Croteau DL, Bohr VA. The role of DNA repair in brain related disease pathology. DNA Repair (Amst). 2013;**12**(8):578-587. DOI: 10.1016/j.dnarep.2013.04.010

[107] Conklin SM, Gianaros PJ, Brown SM, Yao JK, Hariri AR, Manuck SB, et al. Long-chain omega-3 fatty acid intake is associated positively with corticolimbic gray matter volume in healthy adults. Neuroscience Letters. 2007;**421**:209-212. DOI: 10.1016/j.neulet.2007.04.086

[108] Raji CA, Erickson KI, Lopez OL, et al. Regular fish consumption and age-related brain gray matter loss. American Journal of Preventive Medicine. 2014;**47**:444-451. DOI: 10.1016/j.amepre.2014.05.037

[109] Sinn N, Milte CM, Street SJ, Buckley JD, Coates AM, Petkov J, et al. Effects of n-3 fatty acids, EPA v. DHA, on depressive symptoms, quality of life, memory and executive function in older adults with mild cognitive impairment: A 6-month randomised controlled trial. The British Journal of Nutrition. 2012;**107**(11):1682-1693. DOI: 10.1017/S0007114511004788

[110] Miyata J, Arita M. Role of omega-3 fatty acids and their metabolites in asthma and allergic diseases. Allergology International. 2015;**64**(1):27-34. DOI: 10.1016/j.alit.2014.08.003

[111] Kumar A, Mastana SS, Lindley MR. n-3 fatty acids and asthma. Nutrition Research Reviews. 2016;**29**(1):1-16. DOI: 10.1017/S0954422415000116

[112] Yang H, Xun P, He K. Fish and fish oil intake in relation to risk of asthma: A systematic review and meta-analysis. PLoS One. 2013;**8**(11):e80048. DOI: 10.1371/journal.pone.0080048

[113] Li J, Xun P, Zamora D, Sood A, Liu K, Daviglus M, et al. Intakes of long-chain omega-3 (n-3) PUFAs and fish in relation to incidence of asthma among American young adults: The CARDIA study. The American Journal of Clinical Nutrition. 2013;**97**(1):173-178. DOI: 10.3945/ajcn.112.041145. Epub 2012 Nov 28

[114] Bouzianas DG, Bouziana SD, Hatzitolios AI. Potential treatment of human nonalcoholic fatty liver disease with long-chain omega-3 polyunsaturated fatty acids. Nutrition Reviews. 2013;**71**(11):753-771. DOI: 10.1111/nure.12073. Epub 2013 Oct 22

[115] Parker HM, Johnson NA, Burdon CA, Cohn JS, O'Connor HT, George J. Omega-3 supplementation and non-alcoholic fatty liver disease: A systematic review and meta-analysis. Journal of Hepatology. 2012;**56**(4):944-951. DOI: 10.1016/j.jhep.2011.08.018

[116] Burns CP, Halabi S, Clamon G, Kaplan E, Hohl RJ, Atkins JN, et al. Phase II study of high-dose fish oil capsules for patients with cancer-related cachexia. Cancer. 2004;**101**(2):370-378. DOI: 10.1002/cncr.20362

[117] Persson C, Glimelius B, Rönnelid J, Nygren P. Impact of fish oil and melatonin on cachexia in patients with advanced gastrointestinal cancer: A randomized pilot study. Nutrition. 2005;**21**(2):170-178. DOI: 10.1016/j.nut.2004.05.026

[118] Bruera E, Strasser F, Palmer JL, Willey J, Calder K, Amyotte G, et al.

Effect of fish oil on appetite and other symptoms in patients with advanced cancer and anorexia/cachexia: A double-blind, placebo-controlled study. Journal of Clinical Oncology. 2003;**21**(1):129-134. DOI: 10.1200/JCO.2003.01.101

[119] Hamazaki T, Sawazaki S, Itomura M, Asaoka E, Nagao Y, Nishimura N, et al. The effect of docosahexaenoic acid on aggression in young adults. A placebo-controlled double-blind study. The Journal of Clinical Investigation. 1996;**97**(4):1129-1133. DOI: 10.1172/JCI118507

[120] Hamazaki T, Sawazaki S, Nagao Y, Kuwamori T, Yazawa K, Mizushima Y, et al. Docosahexaenoic acid does not affect aggression of normal volunteers under nonstressful conditions. A randomized, placebo-controlled, double-blind study. Lipids. 1998;**33**(7):663-667. DOI: 10.1007/s11745-998-0254-2

[121] Raine A, Portnoy J, Liu J, Mahoomed T, Hibbeln JR. Reduction in behavior problems with omega-3 supplementation in children aged 8-16 years: A randomized, double-blind, placebo-controlled, stratified, parallel-group trial. Journal of Child Psychology and Psychiatry. 2015;**56**(5):509-520. DOI: 10.1111/jcpp.12314. Epub 2014 Aug 22

[122] Xu ZZ, Zhang L, Liu T, Park JY, Berta T, Yang R, et al. Resolvins RvE1 and RvD1 attenuate inflammatory pain via central and peripheral actions. Nature Medicine. 2010;**16**(5):592-597. DOI: 10.1038/nm.2123. 1 p following 597. Epub 2010 Apr 11

[123] Goldberg RJ, Katz J. A meta-analysis of the analgesic effects of omega-3 polyunsaturated fatty acid supplementation for inflammatory joint pain. Pain. 2007;**129**(1-2):210-223. DOI: 10.1016/j.pain.2007.01.020. Epub 2007 Mar 1

[124] Volker D et al. Efficacy of fish oil concentrate in the treatment of rheumatoid arthritis. Journal of Rheumatology. 2000;**27**:2343-2346

[125] Kremer JM. n-3 fatty acid supplements in rheumatoid arthritis. American Journal of Clinical Nutrition. 2000;**71**(suppl):349S-351S

[126] Kruger MC, Horrobin DF. Calcium metabolism, osteoporosis and essential fatty acids: A review. Progress in Lipid Research. 1997;**36**(2-3):131-151

[127] Brusch CA, Et J. A new dietary regimen for arthritis: Value of cod liver oil on a fasting stomach. Journal of the National Medical Association. 1959;**51**(4):266-270 passim

[128] Maggio M, Artoni A, Lauretani F, Borghi L, Nouvenne A, Valenti G, et al. The impact of omega-3 fatty acids on osteoporosis. Current Pharmaceutical Design. 2009;**15**(36):4157-4164. DOI: 10.2174/138161209789909728

[129] Harel Z, Biro FM, Kottenhahn RK, Rosenthal SL. Supplementation with omega-3 polyunsaturated fatty acids in the management of dysmenorrhea in adolescents. American Journal of Obstetrics and Gynecology. 1996;**174**(4):1335-1338. DOI: 10.1016/s0002-9378(96)70681-6

[130] Zafari M, Behmanesh F, Agha MA. Comparison of the effect of fish oil and ibuprofen on treatment of severe pain in primary dysmenorrhea. Caspian Journal of Internal Medicine. 2011;**2**(3):279-282

[131] Ladesich JB, Pottala JV, Romaker A, Harris WS. Membrane level of omega-3 docosahexaenoic acid is associated with severity of obstructive sleep apnea.

Journal of Clinical Sleep Medicine. 2011;**7**(4):391-396. DOI: 10.5664/JCSM.1198

[132] Montgomery P, Burton JR, Sewell RP, Spreckelsen TF, Richardson AJ. Fatty acids and sleep in UK children: Subjective and pilot objective sleep results from the DOLAB study—A randomized controlled trial. Journal of Sleep Research. 2014;**23**(4):364-388. DOI: 10.1111/jsr.12135. Epub 2014 Mar 8

[133] Hansen AL, Dahl L, Olson G, Thornton D, Graff IE, Frøyland L, et al. Fish consumption, sleep, daily functioning, and heart rate variability. Journal of Clinical Sleep Medicine. 2014;**10**(5):567-575. DOI: 10.5664/jcsm.3714

[134] Yamagata K. Docosahexaenoic acid regulates vascular endothelial cell function and prevents cardiovascular disease. Lipids in Health and Disease. 2017;**16**(1):118. DOI: 10.1186/s12944-017-0514-6

[135] Guo XF, Li KL, Li JM, Li D. Effects of EPA and DHA on blood pressure and inflammatory factors: A meta-analysis of randomized controlled trials. Critical Reviews in Food Science and Nutrition. 2019;**59**(20):3380-3393. DOI: 10.1080/10408398.2018.1492901

[136] Stith KR, Ryan AS. The role of docosahexaenoic acid(DHA) in cardiovascular health and sport nutrition, Agro. Food Industry Hi Tech. 2020;**20**(2):59-61

[137] Walser B, Giordano RM, Stebbins CL. Supplementation with omega-3 polyunsaturated fatty acids augments brachial artery dilation and blood flow during forearm contraction. European Journal of Applied Physiology. 2006;**97**(3):347-354. DOI: 10.1007/s00421-006-0190-0

[138] Lalia AZ, Dasari S, Robinson MM, Abid H, Morse DM, Klaus KA, et al. Influence of omega-3 fatty acids on skeletal muscle protein metabolism and mitochondrial bioenergetics in older adults. Aging (Albany NY). 2017;**9**(4):1096-1129. DOI: 10.18632/aging.101210

[139] Ferguson EJ, Seigel JW, McGlory C. Omega-3 fatty acids and human skeletal muscle. Current Opinion in Clinical Nutrition and Metabolic Care. 2021;**24**(2):114-119. DOI: 10.1097/MCO.0000000000000723

[140] Jeromson S, Gallagher IJ, Galloway SD, Hamilton DL. Omega-3 fatty acids and skeletal muscle health. Marine Drugs. 2015;**13**(11):6977-7004. DOI: 10.3390/md13116977

[141] McGlory C, Calder PC, Nunes EA. The influence of omega-3 fatty acids on skeletal muscle protein turnover in health, disuse, and disease. Frontiers in Nutrition. 2019;**6**:144. DOI: 10.3389/fnut.2019.00144

[142] Esmaeili V, Shahverdi AH, Moghadasian MH, Alizadeh AR. Dietary fatty acids affect semen quality: A review. Andrology. 2015;**3**(3):450-461. DOI: 10.1111/andr.12024

[143] Poulos A, Darin-Bennett A, White IG. The phospholipid-bound fatty acids and aldehydes of mammalian spermatozoa. Comparative Biochemistry & Physiology. 1973;**B46**:541-549

[144] Moore HDM. Contribution of epididymal factors to sperm maturation and storage. Andrologia. 1998;**30**:233-239

[145] Schisterman EF, Mumford SL, Chen Z, Browne RW, Boyd Barr D,

Kim S, et al. Lipid concentrations and semen quality: The LIFE study. Andrology. 2014;**2**:408-415

[146] Rachelle Herdman, Erectile Dysfunction is helped by Fish Oil Concentrate. Available from: https://doctorherdmanclinic.com/resources/article/mens-health/erectile-dysfunction-fish-oil-concentrate [Accessed: September 14, 2022]

[147] 10 Surprising Benefits of Fish Oil for Hair Growth. Available from: bebodywise.com [Accessed: September 14, 2022]

[148] Lo Van A, Hachem M, Lagarde M, Bernoud-Hubac N. Omega-3 docosahexaenoic acid is a mediator of fate-decision of adult neural stem cells. International Journal of Molecular Sciences. 2019;**20**(17):4240. DOI: 10.3390/ijms20174240

[149] Kang JX, Wan JB, He C. Concise review: Regulation of stem cell proliferation and differentiation by essential fatty acids and their metabolites. Stem Cells. 2014;**32**(5):1092-1098. DOI: 10.1002/stem.1620

Section 3

Dietary Sources

Chapter 5

The Role of Micronutrients and Micronutrient Supplements in Vegetarian and Vegan Diets

Elizabeth Eveleigh, Lisa Coneyworth and Simon Welham

Abstract

Vegetarian and vegan diets are becoming increasingly popular in Western countries. Numerous global nutrition bodies advocate that appropriately planned meat-free diets are suitable for all the life cycle stages. Nutritionally adequate vegetarian and vegan diets may provide substantial health benefits and reduction of disease states. However, many studies have identified that recommendations for certain micronutrients may be harder to achieve when following these diets. Micronutrient deficiencies can cause several serious health issues throughout life if not prevented and treated. The outcomes of micronutrient deficiencies are particularly severe in vulnerable individuals, including pregnant women and children. Given the large number of individuals now selecting to follow a vegetarian or vegan diet, it is important to address the challenge of achieving micronutrient requirements and to identify methods, such as supplementation, to improve micronutrient intakes in vegetarian and vegan groups.

Keywords: vegan, vegetarian, micronutrients, micronutrient deficiencies, minerals, vitamins, supplements

1. Introduction

Global adoption of meat and animal product-free diets is increasing and, in 2021, around 14% of the UK population identified with these dietary preferences [1]. Vegan and vegetarian diets are characterized by varying levels of restriction of animal products and are recognized by different definitions (**Table 1**). Other subculture diets exist under the definitions of vegetarian and vegan categories. Subcultures are the groups with identities that differ from the dominant culture. In the context of vegan/vegetarian diets, subculture diets are described as those diets that share common dietary restrictions, for example, these do not consume meat but vary slightly from the primary definitions [2]. These include macrobiotic, raw, and fruitarian [2]. Variations in these classifications are significant when discussing the nutritional influence of vegetarian and vegan diets [2].

In 1847, the first vegetarian society was established in the UK [3, 4]. Later, in 1944, the term "vegan" was coined [4]. In the mid-twentieth century, definitions of

Type[1]	Definition
Flexitarian	Occasionally excludes meat and poultry but remains consumption of fish, eggs and dairy
Pescatarian	Excludes meat and poultry but remains consumption of fish, eggs and dairy
Lacto-ovo vegetarian	Excludes meat, poultry and fish but remains consumption of dairy and eggs
Lacto vegetarian	Excludes meat, poultry, fish and eggs but remains consumption of dairy
Ovo vegetarian	Excludes meat, poultry, fish and dairy but remains consumption of eggs
Vegan	Excludes all animal products (meat, poultry, fish, eggs and dairy)

[1]*Diet definitions from Phillips 2004 [2].*

Table 1.
Definition of common vegetarian and vegan diet types.

vegetarian and vegan diets were homogeneous and consisted of those who did not consume animal products (vegans) and those who also may consume dairy and eggs (vegetarians) [2, 4]. Subtypes of the vegetarian diet were later classified based on the type of animal product chosen to consume (**Table 1**) [2]. At this time, individuals were typically consuming "traditional" vegetarian or vegan diets characterized by the intake of vegetables, fruits, beans, legumes, nuts, and seeds [5]. Descriptions of vegetarian and vegan diets further expanded in the 1960s and 1970s with influence from across cultures and religions [4]. In the 1970s and 1980s, micronutrients unfortified milk-alternative beverages and products mimicking meat became more readily available further diversifying vegetarian and vegan diets [4].

In many areas of the world, vegetarian and vegan diets are frequently adopted due to the low availability of animal foods and/or for monetary or religious reasons [6]. In western nations, individuals typically choose to follow vegetarian and vegan diets voluntarily or may adopt them due to food aversion, food allergies, or intolerances [7]. Adherence to vegetarian and vegan diets in Western countries often goes beyond food choice and is closely related to social identity [8]. The top motivations for following vegetarian and vegan diets are ethical and health reasons [9–12]. Ethical motives include environmental and animal welfare concerns in relation with the production of animal-based foods [9, 10]. Health motives often involve the promise of improved health outcomes, weight loss, and reduction of chronic disease states [9, 10]. However, many studies have shown that the adoption of vegan and vegetarian diets may be due to a combination of different motives [9–14]. The acceptance of dietary preferences among family and friends may also influence the uptake of vegetarian and vegan diets [5]. Population subgroups, such as young adults and women, are more likely to adhere to vegetarian and vegan diets [2].

A growing number of people in Western countries are reducing their meat consumption or pledging to follow short-term stints of meat-free diets for campaigns such as Veganuary or Meatless Monday [15, 16]. The rising interest in plant-based eating has amplified demand for commercially available alternative products and convenience items suitable for vegetarians and vegans [17]. Fast-food chains have designed products targeting vegetarian and vegan consumers [18]. Restaurants have expanded menu options to suit all dietary requirements, including an array of vegetarian and vegan products [18]. Additionally, dietary supplements have become more acceptable and available to consumers of vegetarian and vegan diets [19]. It is the position of the British Dietetic Association (BDA), and other societies worldwide, that appropriately planned vegetarian and vegan diets are healthful, nutritionally adequate, and suitable for all stages in the lifecycle, including pregnancy, lactation, infancy, childhood, adolescence, older adulthood, and athletes [20]. However, multiple studies have identified that the restrictive nature of vegetarian and vegan diets may act as a barrier to achieving adequate intake of certain micronutrients, including vitamin B12, vitamin D, iron, zinc, calcium, iodine, and selenium [21–28].

Many plant foods are naturally lower in certain micronutrients in comparison with animal foods and plant-based alternative products are often not fortified with micronutrients to levels equivalent to those found in their animal counterparts [29–32]. Some micronutrients, such as vitamin B12, are only provided by animal products, therefore, vegans and vegetarians with stricter restrictions must rely on fortified foods and/or supplements to achieve optimal B12 intake [33]. Calcium and other micronutrients can only be obtained in small quantities from plant foods, again resulting in reliance on other sources [34]. Furthermore, many micronutrients from plant sources (including iron and zinc) have lower bioavailability due in part to the presence of antinutrients, such as phytates and oxalates, found in whole grains, legumes, and spinach, which impair uptake [35–37]. All these factors may contribute to lowered micronutrient intake and status in individuals following vegetarian or vegan diets.

Modern-day vegetarians and vegans are much more heterogeneous than in the past. Individuals now have a more diverse pool of foods to choose from that are suitable for their dietary preferences, permitting huge variations in food and micronutrient intake. Four distinct dietary patterns within the definition of a vegan diet in UK vegans have been identified [38]. These dietary patterns were termed "convenience" "health conscious," "unhealthy," and "traditional." The least common diet pattern observed was the "traditional" vegan pattern comparable to the vegan diets followed in the 1980s [39]. Although there is yet to be an analysis of the patterns within the vegetarian diet, this suggests that innovation in the vegetarian and vegan food sector is beginning a shift from the healthful "traditional" diet. This change in eating could potentially compromise the micronutrient quality of vegetarian and vegan diets and risk micronutrient deficiencies if diets are not appropriately planned. For example, ultra-processed items, such as meat alternatives and convenience items, are often not fortified with micronutrients and are not nutritionally similar to the foods they are designed to mimic [29, 40, 41]. Alternative dairy products, such as beverages (soya, oat, rice, etc.) and yogurts, are now regularly fortified with vitamin B12, vitamin D, and calcium [30–32, 42]. However, concerns have been raised that these milk alternative beverages do not contain quantities of iodine comparable to dairy and fortification is not yet mandatory [29, 43]. Health-conscious vegetarians and vegans limiting their intake of convenience foods may miss out on the benefits of micronutrient fortification in these products [38]. Moreover, preoccupation with "healthy" eating and inflexibility in the diet has been shown to act as a barrier to micronutrient intake [38]. Supplement usage in vegetarian and vegan populations is variable but can be an efficient way of achieving micronutrient intake [44–47].

Given that these diets are likely to only increase in popularity as we move to more sustainable plant-based diets globally [48, 49], it is paramount to understand the impact of following a vegetarian or vegan diet on micronutrient intake and status to prevent an increase in health problems associated with deficiency. In this chapter, we outline the current literature in this field and discuss the complex issue of obtaining adequate micronutrient intake for those adhering to vegetarian and vegan diets and how this has changed in recent times.

2. Micronutrients

Micronutrients are essential vitamins and minerals required to orchestrate a large proportion of biochemical functions within the body [50]. Most must be supplied in the diet and consequently specific dietary recommendations have been established for each micronutrient by country of origin, age, and sex [51]. In the UK, these recommendations are called Reference Nutrient Intakes (RNIs) [51]. The RNI value for a nutrient is the amount of that nutrient that is sufficient for 97.5% of the population of interest [51]. Lack of adequate provision of micronutrients from the diet can result in micronutrient deficiencies [50]. Although clinical deficiency states are relatively rare in Western countries, mild deficiencies can result in pathological and metabolic changes [50]. In the short-term, undesirable symptoms may occur, which may lead to more severe consequences long-term and potentially even death [52]. Single micronutrient deficiencies are easy to recognize and treat; however, subclinical deficiency states where multiple micronutrients are depleted are more serious and can result in severe complications [52].

3. Key micronutrients over the life cycle

Restrictive diets can pose a risk of micronutrient deficiency during all stages of life, however, the consequences of micronutrient deficiencies are often more serious during periods critical for growth and development (e.g., infancy and pregnancy) [6, 52, 53]. Here, we describe the key micronutrients over the human life cycle.

3.1 Infants and young children (0: 4 years)

There is debate as to whether vegetarian and vegan diets are suitable for infants and young children, for deficiencies of nutrients at this stage of life could have irreversible neurological and developmental consequences [54–60]. Micronutrients, such as iron, zinc, selenium, calcium, and vitamins A, D, and B12, may be problematic in these age groups [54–59, 61]. Infants and children tend to consume diets chosen by their caregivers [2]; therefore, achieving micronutrient intake is subject to the nutritional knowledge of the food provider. Micronutrient consumption may therefore be impaired if strict ideologies and food choices are imposed [2].

In the UK, exclusive breastfeeding (feeding only breast milk) is promoted for the first 6 months of infancy [62]. The maternal diet influences the nutrient composition of breast milk, particularly B vitamins and vitamins A, C, and D [63]. Breast milk typically has low quantities of vitamin D, it is now recommended that all breastfed infants consume a vitamin D supplement of 8.5–10 mg day^{-1} [64]. Generally, exclusively breastfed vegetarian children do not struggle to meet micronutrient requirements [6]; however, vegan and vegetarian mothers have been shown to produce milk with lower vitamin B12 concentrations [6], so B12 must be considered when vegetarian or vegan mothers select to exclusively breastfeed [6]. Studies of UK vegans have also found breast milk riboflavin content to be lower than omnivorous participants [65]. Riboflavin has a significant role as a co-enzyme in energy metabolism (flavin mononucleotide (FMN) and flavin adenine dinucleotide (FAD)) [66]. Riboflavin deficiency is not fatal but can cause clinical symptoms after several months of inadequate intake (RNI by age: 0–6 months; < 0.3 mg, 7–12 months; < 0.4 mg, 1–3 years; < 0.5 mg) [51]. Mild symptoms of riboflavin deficiency include sore throat and loss of hair [66]. Whereas anemia and impaired nerve functioning may present in more severe deficiency states [66]. Infants that are not breastfed before 1 year of age are recommended to consume commercially available infant formulas [67]. Formulas are usually made from modified cow's milk [67] and are not appropriate for infants following a vegan diet. Infant formula made of methionine-fortified soya protein isolate is available for infants with cow's milk allergy [67]. Infant formula milk is typically fortified with vitamins A, C, and D, but there are currently no vegan formulas available in the UK in part because vitamin D fortification is dependent on lanolin from sheep's wool [64]. Soya formula has been extensively studied to ensure that infants grow and develop correctly. Studies have found no difference in infant development-fed soya formula compared to cow's milk formula [68]. Cow's milk and soya milk are not recommended prior to the first year of life as iron concentration and bioavailability are too low to meet requirements for growth [67]. Soya milk also has a low zinc concentration and bioavailability [69]. Nutritional concerns have been raised for vegetarian and vegan infants who have been given homemade plant milks (e.g., oat, soya, etc.), vegetable or fruit juices, or milks not recommended for individuals in the first year of life [70].

In the UK, infants can be introduced to solid foods (complementary feeding or weaning) at 6 months of age [71]. Advice for weaning is the same for vegetarian and vegan infants as for infants following an omnivorous diet [71]. Iron, calcium, zinc, iodine, and vitamin D and B12 must be carefully considered for weaning infants [57]. In infancy, vitamin D and calcium are essential for bone growth and bone mass attainment, whereas, iron, zinc, and iodine deficiency can have potential neurodevelopmental implications [70]. After 1 year, vegetarian and vegan infants can be weaned onto suitable diets containing cow's milk or fortified (vitamin B12, D, and calcium) soy-based milk [57, 70, 71]. If fortified variants are not available, then micronutrient supplements (vitamins B12 and D) must be considered [72]. In 2021, there was a call for evidence in the UK to assess if dairy-free infant formulas should be mandatorily fortified with iodine (for infants 0–5 years) as these products contain lower quantities compared to cow's milk-based products [73].

Young children, aged 1–4 years, experience large variations in growth rates, dietary patterns, and nutrient losses, making it difficult to assess micronutrient requirements and intake [58]. Studies have found that iron, calcium, and vitamin D intake tends to be lower in vegan children compared to vegetarian and omnivorous children [58]. Parents of vegan and vegetarian infants and young children may wish to seek support from a General Practitioner (GP) or Registered Dietician to ensure that micronutrient recommendations are achieved.

3.2 Childhood (4: 13 years)

Childhood is characterized by the rapid development of cognitive and physical function; therefore, sufficient micronutrient intake is critical [74]. Iron, zinc, vitamin D, iodine, calcium, and particularly vitamin B12, all have roles in growth and development at this stage [74]. Iron and zinc are particularly important in pubertal vegetarian and vegan girls, for menstruation losses to be replenished [75], while calcium and vitamin D are important for bone growth and metabolism [76]. Many cereals and alternative foods are now fortified with these key micronutrients and should be available to growing children by parents or caregivers [60, 77, 78]. At the time of this publication, there is limited research investigating vegan and vegetarian diets and micronutrient intake in childhood [78]. From the available research, childhood vegan diets have been reported to be lower in micronutrients required for optimal bone health cobalamin, calcium, and vitamin D. A study in 2021 found that vegan children aged 5–10 years tend to be shorter by 3 cm and have 4–6% lower bone mineral mass compared to omnivorous children [79]. Similarly, B12 intake was found to be lower in this particular study [79]. Adequate intake of micronutrients at this age is therefore essential to reduce the risk of fractures and potentially osteoporosis in later life [79].

3.3 Adolescents and young adults (14–25 years)

Adolescents and young adults (14–25 years) have more autonomy in their food choices, and this is typically the life stage where eating behaviors are adopted [80]. Adolescents may transition to a vegetarian or vegan diet as an expression of identity [8]. Adolescence is typically characterized by poor diet quality [81], especially for students and vegetarian or vegan individuals, increased consumption of unfortified and heavily processed vegan junk foods may limit the intake of iron, zinc, vitamin D, vitamin B12, iodine, and calcium [38]. Another concern is that adolescents may adopt vegetarian or vegan diets to mask eating disorders, further increasing the risk of inadequate micronutrient intake [82, 83]. This potentially poses a greater risk as young women approach childbearing years [28, 84–86]. For women of childbearing age, a well-planned diet prior to conception is essential for fertility and the maintenance of healthy pregnancy [87]. Women of childbearing age are consequently recommended to consume supplements during pre-conception and pregnancy to meet increased micronutrient requirements [87].

3.4 Pregnancy and lactation

Nutritional requirements increase to support maternal metabolism and tissue formation, along with fetal growth and development [87]. Supplementation of iron, zinc, folic acid, vitamin D, iodine, and B vitamins may be more necessary in individuals following vegetarian or vegan diets as inadequate micronutrient intake is more frequent [88]. In the UK, pregnant women are able to apply for free vitamin tablets as part of the NHS Healthy Start Scheme, which contain folic acid that lowers the chance of babies having spinal problems, vitamin C, and vitamin D [89]. The Healthy Start Scheme also provides cash cards for low-income households to buy certain types of milk, infant formula, fruit, and vegetables [89]. Adoption of a well-planned and micronutrient-rich diet is essential in pregnancy [6]. If achieved, pregnancy outcomes are no different from that reported in omnivorous individuals [6]. Individuals following vegetarian and vegan diets during pre-conception and pregnancy may benefit from direct support from health professionals as a preventative measure to ensure dietary recommendations are achieved [6]. Moreover, dietary behaviors adopted during pregnancy and post-pregnancy influence food choices and preferences of future offspring, which can have lifelong impacts on the child's eating habits and micronutrient intake [6].

3.5 Adulthood (18: 60 years)

In adulthood and mid-life, micronutrients are required in adequate quantities to diminish the age-related cognitive and physical decline in later life [81]. Vegetarian and vegan adults may be at risk of deficiencies, including vitamin B12, vitamin D, iron, zinc, calcium, iodine, and selenium [81]. If individuals adopt vegetarian and vegan diets to lose weight, then inadequate food provision may further limit micronutrient intake if not balanced appropriately [24, 90, 91].

3.6 Elderly and old age (60+ years)

Elderly populations have lower requirements for most micronutrients as physical and metabolic demands are reduced [92]. However, they often exhibit deficiencies in folic acid, vitamin D, calcium, selenium, and vitamin B12 [92]. Older adults living in institutions, who are frail or overweight, consequently have a higher risk of micronutrient deficiency [92]. Additional barriers to achieving micronutrient intake in old age include limited ability to purchase food, poverty, loss of taste or smell, infections, and other diseases, such as dementia and drug interactions [93]. Micronutrient deficiencies may also be more common in elderly populations because of gastrointestinal complaints that reduce the absorption of fat-soluble vitamins [93]. Deficiencies may also occur due to a lack of diet diversity [92]. Frail elderly populations may be unable to cook for themselves, becoming reliant on ready meals and processed food items that are palatable and easy to prepare [92]. At present, the approximate number of elderly people following a vegan or vegetarian diet is unknown. In 2021, it was estimated that 1/5 of vegans in the UK are above the age of 40 years and are heading toward old age [94]. There is expected to be an increase in the number of elderly vegans and vegetarians in the coming years given the rise in popularity of these diets and the global shift to more sustainable diets. Whilst, there is little research covering micronutrients in elderly vegetarians and vegans, dependence on unfortified vegetarian and vegan convenience items, and disuse or avoidance of dietary supplements may further reduce micronutrient intake [43]. It is therefore important to promote the consumption of fortified foods and dietary supplements for the elderly who select to follow a vegetarian or vegan diet.

4. Prevalence of micronutrient deficiencies in adulthood

The study of micronutrients in vegetarian and vegan diets is a rapidly evolving field of nutrition, advanced in accordance with the global recognition of these diets. Much of the nutritional evidence focusing on these diets were collected in the 1980s [5]. In this section, we will address the prevalence of micronutrient deficiencies in the "second wave" vegetarian and vegan movement supported today (2010–2022).

4.1 Vitamin deficiencies

Adult (19–50 years) RNIs for key vitamins, their function, and symptoms of deficiency are shown in **Table 2** [51]. Vitamins are classified into two groups according to their solubility [96]. Water-soluble vitamins (B vitamins and C) diffuse freely in plasma and cytoplasm, are not easily stored, and are excreted in urine [96]. Fat-soluble vitamins include vitamins A, D, E, and K which, once absorbed [97], are retained for longer than water-soluble vitamins.

4.1.1 Water-soluble vitamins

Water-soluble vitamins need a constant regular intake to prevent deficiency [96]. Deficiencies in water-soluble vitamins B2, Niacin, and B12 are common in vegetarian and vegan diets [98].

Vitamin	RNI[1]	Functions[2]	Symptoms of deficiency[2]
A (Retinol, β-Carotene)	Male; 700.0 μg Female; 600.0 μg	Regulator of gene expression and cell differentiation, creation of pigments in the retina for vision and antioxidant capacity	Night blindness (Xerophthalmia) and skin keratinization
D (Calciferol)	10.0 μg	Controls calcium balance, involved in bone mineralization and intestinal absorption of calcium (Ca^{2+})	Rickets and Osteomalacia both related to bone mineralization.
E (Tocopherols, Tocotrienols)	Male; 4 mg Female; 3 mg	Antioxidant capacity	(Rare) Neurological dysfunction
K (Phylloquinone, Menaquinones)	1 μg per kg body weight	Coenzyme required for formation of proteins used in blood clotting and bone formation	Disorders of blood clotting
B1 (Thiamin)	Male; 1.0 mg Female; 0.8 mg	Coenzyme used in nerve transmission	Peripheral nerve damage (Beri beri) and central nervous system dysfunction (Wernicke-Korsakoff syndrome)
B2 (Riboflavin)	Male; 1.3 mg Female; 1.1 mg	Coenzyme used in cellular growth and function by oxidation and reduction reactions	Injury to corner of mouth, lips and tongue (debhorroeic dermatitis)
Niacin (Nicotinic Acid, Nicotinamide)	Male; 16.4 mg Female; 13.2 mg	Coenzyme in oxidation and reduction reactions that produce energy for cells	Pellagra
B6 (Pyridoxine, Pyridoxal, Pyridoxamine)	Male; 1.4 mg[3] Female; 1.2 mg[3]	Coenzyme in amino acid and glycogen breakdown and has a role in steroid hormone action	Disorders of amino acid metabolism
B12 (Cobalamin)	1.5 μg	Coenzyme used to form red blood cells, DNA, brain and nerve cells. Also used in the metabolism of folate	Pernicious anemia (deficiency in production of red blood cells) and degradation of the spinal cord.
Folic Acid (Folate)	200 μg	Coenzyme used in cell development and metabolism such as the conversion of homocysteine to methionine and specific anticonvulsant drugs	Megaloblastic anemia (production of unusually large, immature red blood cells called megablasts)
C (Ascorbic Acid)	40 mg	Coenzyme with antioxidant functioning which enhances the absorption of iron	Scurvy

[1]*Data provided by the British Nutrition Foundation [51].*
[2]*Information from Introduction to Human Nutrition, 3rd Edition [95].*
[3]*Based on protein providing 14.7% of Estimated Average Requirement (EAR) for energy.*

Table 2.
UK Adult (19–50 years) Reference Nutrient Intake (RNI) for key vitamins, functions, and symptoms of deficiency.

Riboflavin (vitamin B2) is naturally present in a variety of foods and commonly fortified in cereals, thus deficiency is relatively rare [66]. Milk and dairy products are important sources of vitamin B2 in the western diet, and these alongside other animal products contain B2 in greater quantities compared with plant foods [99]. Recent studies have identified absorption of vitamin B2 to be lower in vegans due to both inadequate intake and reduced bioavailability of B2 from non-animal sources [99]. The bioavailability of foods will be discussed in later sections. Further work has identified that 25% of vegans may be deficient in vitamin B2 compared to 14% of omnivores [99].

Niacin is present in fish and meat, along with fortified foods such as cereals, legumes, and bread [95]. Small quantities can also be synthesized internally from the dietary amino acid tryptophan, but not at an amount to satisfy daily requirements. Several plant foods contain niacin in the form of niacin–glycosides, where niacin is bound to sugar molecules [100]. These are common in grains such as wheat and corn [100]. In this form, the bioavailability of niacin is diminished and may even be prevented altogether. Individuals reliant on plant foods therefore may find it more challenging to access niacin [100–102]. Moreover, individuals with low diet diversity and an over-reliance on wheat and corn may find it more challenging to meet requirements [100]. Studies have shown that vegans typically have the lowest intake of niacin, compared to other dietary groups, and may not be able to achieve recommendations [98].

Vitamin B12 (Cobalamin) is only provided in substantial quantities by the consumption of animal and dairy products, therefore adequate intake by individuals following vegan diets is dependent on the consumption of fortified foods, including cereals, soy or dairy alternatives (beverages, yogurts, etc.) along with supplements or food additives (e.g., nutritional yeast) [103]. Inadequate intake of vitamin B12 is common in vegan and vegetarian diets. Blood biomarkers, including serum cobalamin, can be used to assess vitamin B12 status [104]. A systematic review investigating blood serum concentration of Cobalamin (Cbl) in vegetarian adults and older adults found that deficiency was present in up to 86.5% of individuals [105, 106]. Further research identified longer-term vegans are more likely to experience vitamin B12 deficiency due to the depletion of bodily stores over time [105, 106]. Folic acid deficiency can occur consequent to vitamin B12 deficiency due to impaired methionine synthase action [107]. Methionine synthase is responsible for the restoration of methionine from homocysteine, inhibition of this enzyme traps folate as methyl tetrahydrofolate [107]. This phenomenon is called the "Folate trap" [107].

4.1.2 Fat-soluble vitamins

Vitamin D has been recorded to be significantly lower in vegetarian and vegan diets compared to omnivores [98]. Vitamin D can be endogenously generated via skin exposure to the sun [108–110]. Therefore, status does largely depend on non-food-related factors, including skin color, season, geographical location, duration of sun exposure, and quantity of sun exposure [108–111]. Dietary sources of vitamin D are limited and are, for the most part, animal products [111]. Vitamin D increases the intestinal efficacy of calcium and phosphate absorption for proper formation of the bone mineral matrix [76, 108, 109]. Deficiency may therefore lead to reduced calcium absorption and heighten the risk of developing osteomalacia and other bone disorders [76, 108, 109]. Regardless of dietary preference, vitamin D deficiency is a UK-wide issue, recently around one in five adults have been identified as having levels of vitamin D in their blood (circulating 25(OH)D) corresponding to deficiency (< 25 nmol L^{-1}) [110].

Other vitamin deficiencies are uncommon in vegetarian and vegan diets due to greater consumption of plant foods compared to omnivores [99].

4.2 Mineral deficiencies

Adult (19–50 years) RNIs for each mineral, function, and symptoms of deficiency are shown in **Table 3** [51]. Minerals can be grouped according to the quantity required in the body [95]. Calcium, phosphorus, and magnesium are vital in large amounts and are known as macrominerals [95]. Minerals needed in smaller amounts are called trace elements (iron, zinc, fluoride, selenium, copper, chromium, and iodine) [95]. Trace elements may be nutritionally essential or nonessential. All trace elements can be toxic if consumed in excess for long time periods [95].

4.2.1 Macrominerals

Calcium has been identified as a problem micronutrient in vegetarian and vegan diets as it is less bioavailable from plant foods than from animal sources [95]. Absorption is limited in plant foods by inhibiting substances oxalate, phytate, and dietary fiber [95]. Water is, however, a valuable source of dietary calcium and can be consumed by all diet types, and many food products targeted at vegetarians and vegans, including alternative milk beverages, yogurts, and spreads, are now fortified with calcium [31, 32, 42, 112]. Despite this, calcium intake tends to be lowest in vegans compared with non-vegans, and a recent systematic review showed that 76% of vegan participants had intakes that were less than the RNI for calcium [98]. Additional studies investigating blood plasma calcium levels show that vegans have significantly lower plasma calcium concentrations compared to non-vegans and a growing number of papers indicate that vegans and vegetarians are at increased risk of bone fractures and bone disorders in later life [34, 113, 114].

4.2.2 Trace elements

Dietary iron comprises two forms, haem and non-haem ferric (Fe^{3+}) iron [115, 116]. Only haem iron and reduced ferrous (Fe^{2+}) iron are absorbed [115, 116]; haem iron via the heam transporter and Fe^{2+} via the divalent metal transporter 1 (DMT1) present on the apical membrane of the small intestinal epithelial cell (enterocyte) [115, 116]. Plant foods only contain non-haem iron which must be converted to $Fe2^{+}$ and consequently, is less effectively absorbed compared with haem iron. Fe^{3+} is reduced to Fe^{2+} via the ferric reductase enzyme duodenal cytochrome B (Dcytb) which oxidizes vitamin C in the process [115]. Non-haem is rendered less bioavailable because its absorption i additionally inhibited by naturally occurring molecules such as phytate, oxalate, and polyphenols [95]. The Institute of Medicine has stated that iron requirements for vegetarians should be 1.8x greater than omnivores for this reason [117]. Recent studies have suggested that vegans may have greater iron intakes than other dietary groups, but the elevated level may still not be sufficient to overcome the bioavailability issues [118, 119]. In support of this, circulating ferritin, a biomarker of iron availability, is low in vegans [118]. Some studies have failed to show that vegetarians and vegans are any

Mineral	RNI[1]	Functions[2]	Symptoms of deficiency[2]
Calcium	700 mg	Required for growth and skeletal formation, muscle contraction, membrane transport and signal transduction	Hypocalcemia, Osteopenia and Osteoporosis
Phosphorus	550 mg[3]	Structural component of bones and teeth and DNA/RNA and contributes to bipolarity of lipid membranes and lipoproteins, with metabolic functions e.g. signal transduction and gene transcription.	Hypophosphatemia and non-nutritional cause of Rickets and Osteomalacia
Magnesium	Male; 300 mg Female; 270 mg	Cofactor in energy metabolism, synthetizes of carbohydrates, lipids, nucleic acids, proteins and bone development	Reduced plasma and red blood cell magnesium, Hypocalcemia. Hypocalciuria and Hypokalemia
Sodium	1600 mg[4]	Regulation of osmotic and electrolyte balance involved in nerve conduction, cellular transport and formation of bone	Hyponatremia
Potassium	3500 mg[5]	Intra cellular fluid regulation, muscle contraction and blood pressure regulation	Hypokalemia
Chloride	2500 mg[6]	Intra cellular fluid regulation, muscle contraction, blood pressure regulation and balance of pH	Hypochloremia and metabolic alkalosis
Iron	Male; 8.7 mg Female; 14.8 mg[7]	Blood cell and hormone production and cofactor for enzymes involved in oxidative phosphorylation	Iron deficiency anemia
Zinc	Male; 9.5 mg Female; 7.0 mg	DNA and protien synthesis, cell growth, tissue and cell repair, and immune function	Bullous-pustular dermatitis, alopecia, diarrhea, mood disorders, weight loss, infections and male hypogonadism
Copper	1.2 mg	Growth, cardiovascular and lung integrity, neovascularization, neuroendocrine function, and iron metabolism.	Hypocupremia, anemia (microcytic, normocytic, or macrocytic), neutropenia, thrombocytopenia and myelopathy and peripheral neuropathy
Selenium	Male; 75 μg Female; 60 μg	Component of selenoproteins performing metabolic functions e.g. thyroid hormone activation and immune system functioning	Cardiovascular disease, infertility, myodegenerative diseases, and cognitive decline
Iodine	140 μg	Component of the thyroid hormones regulating growth and metabolism	Hypothyroidism, goiter cretinism (infants only), and impaired cognitive development (infants only)

[1]*Data provided by the British Nutrition Foundation [51].*
[2]*Information from Introduction to Human Nutrition, 3rd Edition [95].*
[3]*Phosphorous RNI is equal to calcium in molar terms.*
[4]*1 mmol sodium = 23 mg.*
[5]*1 mmol potassium = 39 mg.*
[6]*Corresponds to sodium 1 mmol = 35.5.*
[7]*Insuffcent recommendation for individuals with high menstrual losses, iron supplements may be required.*

Table 3.
UK Adult (19–50 years) Reference Nutrient Intake (RNI) for key minerals, functions, and symptoms of deficiency.

more likely to develop iron deficiency anemia than omnivores, however, young women adhering to vegetarian and vegan diets tend to have blood hemoglobin (Hb) concentrations that are indicative of anemia [118].

Many recent studies have identified that intakes of iodine within vegan and vegetarian populations are suggestive of mild to severe deficiency [25, 27, 28]. Individuals following omnivorous diets tend to have significantly greater iodine intake [26], as iodine is found in fish, seafood, eggs, and dairy products [120]. Plant foods have a low iodine concentration, and their iodine content is dependent on the content of the soil in which it has been grown [121]. However, even in high iodine areas, plants contain very low levels as it is not actively absorbed [122]. Across much of the globe, salt is mandatorily fortified with iodine (iodized salt), but this is not so in the UK, hence the capacity for individuals living in the UK to achieve dietary adequacy is more limited without the consumption of animal products and is reliant upon supplements or fortified foods which are limited in number [123, 124].

A small number of studies have found selenium intake to be significantly lower in vegan diets compared to vegetarians [28, 125]. Vegetarians can consume selenium from dairy products, such as eggs, yogurt, cheese, and milk [95], whilst vegans may be more vulnerable to selenium deficiency because of excluding them from the diet [28]. A recent exploratory study in the UK found that selenium intake was below the lower RNI of 50% [28]. Both selenium and iodine are found in similar foods and are linked to thyroid hormone production and thyroid hormone action [126]. These deficiencies are often coupled and can exert similar deficiency states [126].

5. Characteristics potentiating micronutrient deficiencies

As with all diets, there are certain factors that may increase the risk of micronutrient deficiencies.

5.1 Diet

Diet is the main component that needs to be considered when evaluating the adequacy of vegetarian/vegan diets. Individuals following diets with less extensive avoidance of animal products or those that eat larger quantities of fish, seafood, dairy products, and/or eggs are likely to have improved micronutrient intake [98]. Individuals with greater restrictions must consume other micronutrient-rich foods, fortified foods, or dietary supplements [2]. A select proportion of individuals may choose to further avoid fortified foods, dietary supplements, and processed alternatives due to personal, ideological, or religious reasons [2]. Additional avoidance of specific food items, for example, only eating raw or organic foods or experiencing food neophobia may further risk micronutrient deficiency [2].

Food consumption may also be limited for involuntary reasons. Individuals living in urban areas may have better availability and access to specialist vegetarian and vegan foods and food outlets compared to those living in smaller rural areas [127]. Similarly, there may be a lack of suitable supplements and fortified foods to meet requirements for certain micronutrients [29]. The price of vegetarian and vegan foods may further act as a barrier to achieving adequate micronutrient intake [127]. Socio-economic status may therefore further influence food intake and availability [127].

5.2 Bioavailability and absorption of micronutrients

The European Food Information Council (EUFIC) describes bioavailability as "the proportion of a nutrient that is absorbed from the diet and used for normal body functions" [128]. Consumed food is digested and absorbed in the intestine. The bioavailability of micronutrients in different food stuffs is affected by various factors (**Table 4**) [35]. Plant foods tend to have significantly lower bioavailability of micronutrients compared to animal products.

5.3 Health status

Micronutrient status is linked to health status and age. Life stages that require rapid growth (fetus, infant, children, and those going through puberty) as well as pregnant and lactating women who need to support rapid growth, need greater micronutrient intake [52]. Individuals who are gaining weight and are experiencing rapid anabolism (e.g., bodybuilders and regular gym goers) or those with high energy requirements for exercise have greater requirements [52]. Diseases such as anorexia and chronic alcohol misuse, digestive diseases, and intolerances or allergies reduce food intake and consequently micronutrient intake along with any condition that causes unintentional weight loss of more than 5% of weight per month [52]. Individuals with increased requirements for metabolism caused by surgery, infection, or trauma will demand a greater supply of water-soluble vitamins (vitamins B and C) and minerals [52]. Loss of body fluids leads to a reduction in micronutrient stores [52]. This may be from excessive diuresis (either from disease or consumption of diuretic drugs), hemorrhage (menstruation or trauma), or diarrhea [52].

5.4 Personal characteristics and beliefs

Deeply ingrained philosophical, ethical, or religious beliefs may dictate food choices and may not be planned according to nutritional recommendations provided by expert bodies [2]. Vegetarianism and veganism are strongly linked with a number of religions, including Hindus, Buddhists, Rastafarians, Seventh-Day Adventists, and Jains [5]. Seventh-Day Adventists following a lacto-ovo vegetarian diet are among those who make a conscious effort to follow the guidance of nutritional professionals and are often

- Gender
- Age and life stage (e.g. pregnancy/children)
- Body composition
- Health status
- Nutrient status
- Structure of foods
- Cooking and processing
- Chemical form of micronutrients
- Interactions between micronutrients
- Non micronutrient inhibitors and enhancers (factors that decrease/increase absorption)

Table 4.
Factors influencing the bioavailability of micronutrients.

used in epidemiological studies of the vegetarian diet [5]. However, some regimes may demonize certain food groups and eating practices or reject nutritional recommendations [2]. Conformity and group pressure may reinforce negative beliefs around food choice [2, 7]. Nutritional knowledge and education are linked to adequate micronutrient status [84, 129–131]. Individuals with good knowledge of how to correctly balance and plan a vegetarian or vegan diet are likely to have more adequate micronutrient intake [25]. Improving knowledge of how to achieve micronutrient recommendations would therefore be beneficial to those choosing to follow vegetarian and vegan diets [25, 28].

6. Achieving micronutrient recommendations for individuals

A well-planned vegetarian or vegan diet can provide an adequate intake of all micronutrients [20]. The UK government advises that a vegetarian diet should be planned according to the Eatwell Guide (**Figure 1**) [132]. The Vegan Society has created a vegan-specific version of the Eatwell Guide to support individuals who choose a diet that excludes animal products (**Figure 2**) [133]. The Eatwell Guide and Vegan Eatwell Guide are divided into sections and are comprised of example foods and portion sizes required for a healthy diet. There is no standard universal healthy diet for those following vegetarian and vegan diets, nevertheless, the Eatwell Guide and Vegan Eatwell Guide direct individuals to consume dietary patterns that include higher consumption of fruit and vegetables, wholegrains, pulses, nuts and seeds, and a lower intake of fatty/processed foods, refined grains, sugar-sweetened foods and beverages, salt, and saturated fat [133].

The Eatwell Guide does not give specific guidance on how to achieve RNI of micronutrients within a vegetarian or vegan diet. Conversely, the guide does include

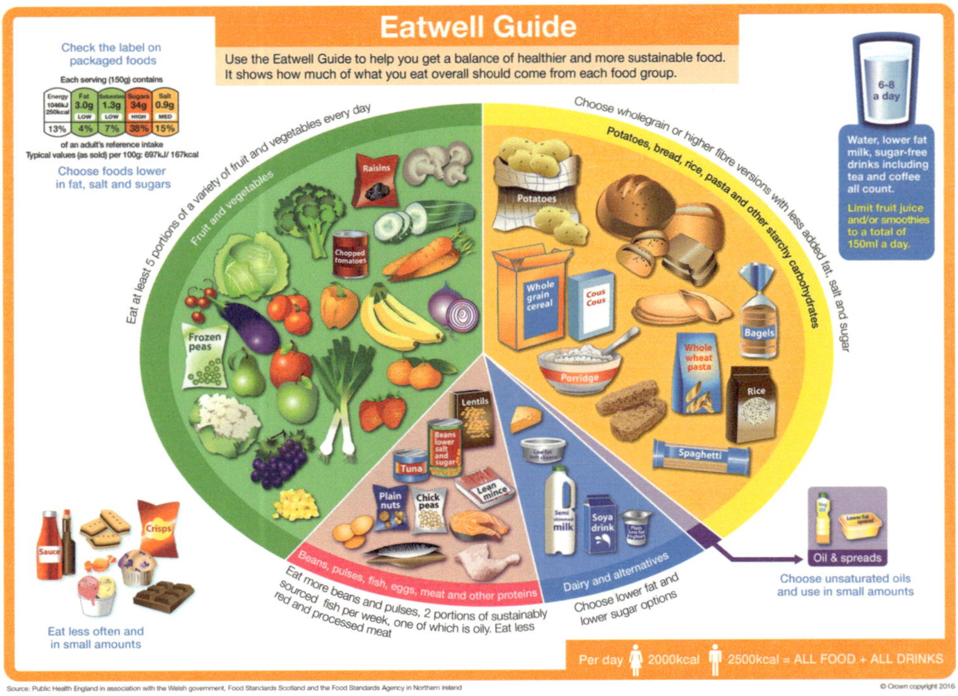

Figure 1.
The Eatwell Guide UK 2016 [132].

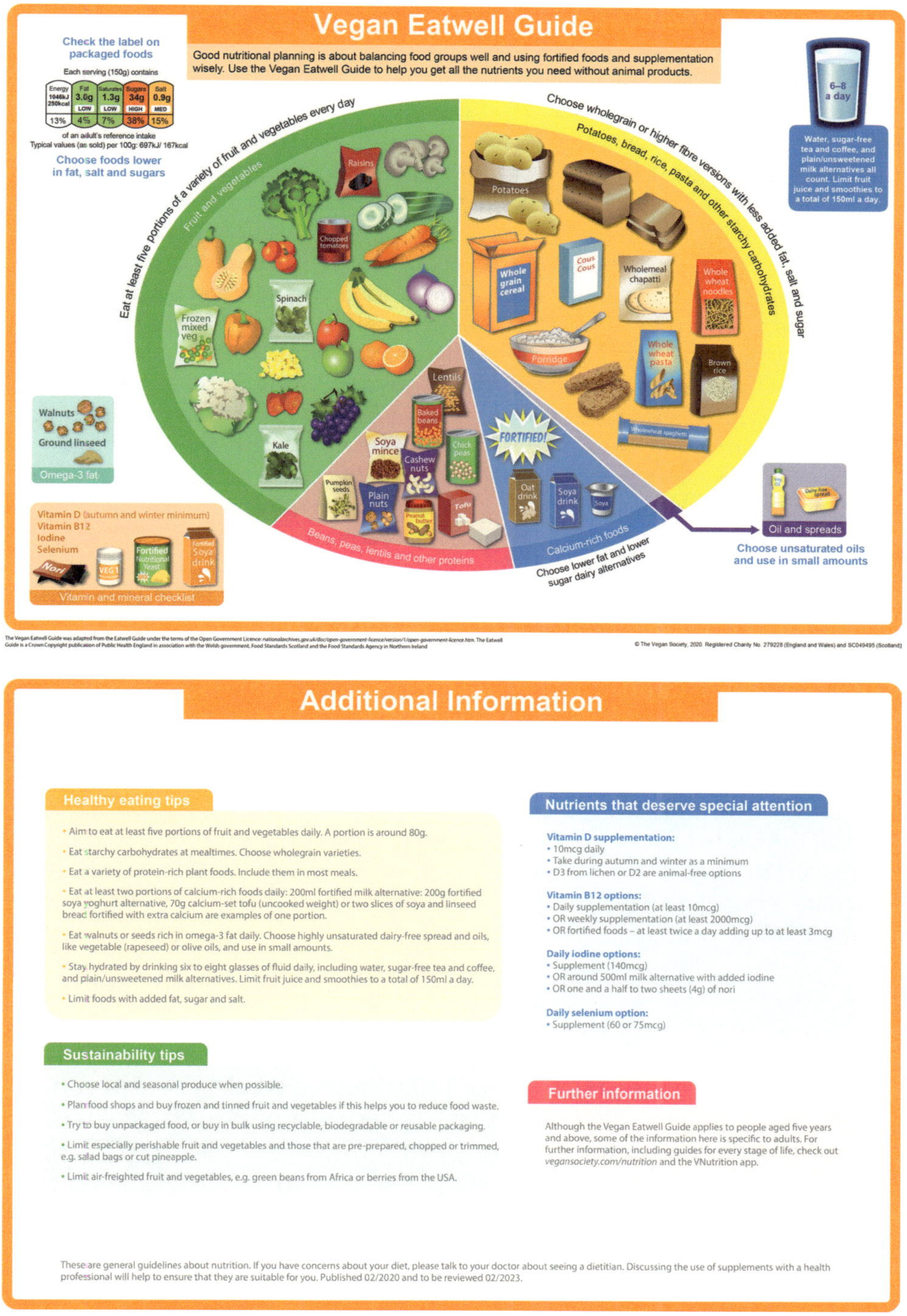

Figure 2.
The Vegan Eatwell Guide adapted from the Eatwell Guide by The Vegan Society 2020 [133].

notes to lead users to select micronutrient-fortified alternative products, sprinkles, and supplements. However, as discussed, without substantial dietary planning certain micronutrients may be missed from vegetarian and vegan diets.

6.1 Consumption of fortified foods

Food fortification describes the process of adding nutrients to foods either to return nutrients that have been lost through processing or to improve the nutrient content of foods [134]. Fortified foods are useful to ensure adequate micronutrient intake when certain food groups are excluded from the diet [134]. In the 1940s, the UK introduced mandatory fortification of white flour with vitamin B2 and other B-complex vitamins to improve its nutrient profile following processing [135]. In 2022, there was a call for evidence launched by the UK Government to identify methods for improving the vitamin D status of the population [136]. Fortification of staple food products, such as cereals and flour, has been identified as a technique to improve vitamin D intake for at-risk population groups, such as vegetarians and vegans [110, 136].

Some vegetarian and vegan-appropriate foods are already fortified with key micronutrients including vitamin D, calcium, and B-complex vitamins, for example, yeast extract, nutritional yeast, grains, cereals, alternative dairy products (e.g., dairy-free cheeses, fat spreads, yogurts, etc.) and alternative milk beverages [133]. Nutritional yeast is a good source of micronutrients providing 6 mg per portion (1 tbsp) of zinc [137]. One serving of fortified alternative milk beverage (200 ml) may provide an average of 1.5 μg of vitamin D, 0.2 mg of B2, 0.76 μg of B12, and 240 mg of calcium (30% of nutrient reference values in the UK) [137]. However, alternative milk beverages fortified with tricalcium phosphate as a method of calcium fortification may not be a like-for-like comparison to cow's milk [137]. Additionally, iodine-fortified milk alternative beverages are also a good source of iodine, with one portion serving at 45 μg per 200 ml. Currently, most alternative milk beverages on the UK market are not iodine fortified [29]. The British Dietetic Association (BDA) is currently petitioning to change the governmental policy around alternative milks to ensure that all are required to be fortified with iodine to be sold in the UK to help improve iodine intake in populations that do not consume cow's milk [138]. Therefore, it is important to check nutrition labels carefully during purchasing of products to ensure the selection of products adequately fortified with micronutrients.

6.1.1 Iodized salt

In many countries worldwide, iodine is added to table salt in the form of potassium iodate or iodide [123, 124]. Universal Salt Iodization (USI) is the most cost-effective and simple route to improving population iodine intake [123, 124]. In the UK, no USI is present and iodized salt is not used in commercial food processing [123]. Iodized salt brands are available to purchase in a very limited number of UK supermarkets [123]. A 1.5 g portion provides approximately 20% of the RNI for iodine [123]. Iodized salt intake must agree to UK recommendations whereby adults should eat no more than 6 g of salt a day [123].

6.1.2 Supplementation

The Food Standards Agency UK defines a supplement as "any food the purpose of which is to supplement the normal diet and which is a concentrated source of a vitamin or mineral or other substance with a nutritional or physiological effect, alone or in combination and is sold in dose form" [139]. Micronutrient supplementation is usually the provision of single or multiple micronutrients in consumable form (capsules, tablets, drops, etc.) with the aim of correcting or maintaining adequate micronutrient intake for optimal human health.

Micronutrient supplements are easily accessible, and being sold in a range of shops including supermarkets, pharmacies, and health shops [140]. Popular micronutrient supplements include vitamins D, C, and B12, along with minerals iron and calcium [140]. Most individuals can achieve adequate micronutrient intake by improving their diet quality, however, the BDA suggests that people following a vegan diet may benefit from taking micronutrient supplements [140].

Information on supplement consumption and its impact on vegans and vegetarians is relatively sparse. A recent systematic review found that only 39% (55/141) of studies assessed the contribution of supplements to dietary micronutrient intake [36]. The authors found that, for the most part, micronutrient intake in vegans did not differ considerably between those whose intake relied exclusively on foods and those who additionally consumed supplements [36]. Vitamin B12 and D were the exceptions to this, whereby intake and status tended to be lower in non-supplementing vegans and vegetarians. Most studies show that individuals following a vegan diet consume supplements more frequently than omnivores [36], particularly those providing B12 [25, 113]. Greater B12 supplementation in vegan populations is likely due to the general awareness that people following a vegan diet have regarding the higher risk of vitamin B12 deficiency [33, 141]. However, it is apparent from other work that awareness of potential deficiencies for other micronutrients such as iodine, is less common [25, 142].

There is still little robust evidence on the supplement intake of vegans and vegetarians in the modern day. This is likely to be due to methodological issues associated with accurate reporting of micronutrient supplements in dietary surveys. Patterns of supplement consumption can vary substantially over a period of time and varies considerably between individuals. The dose and type of supplement consumed differ widely and various other parameters, including life-stage, also need to be considered before introducing supplements to the diet [143]. There is a need for more comprehensive studies of micronutrient supplement use in vegan and vegetarian diets.

In the UK, the population is recommended to consume a daily 10 μg vitamin D supplement between October and March when sun exposure is lower regardless of dietary practice [136, 144]. Studies have identified that the rate of vegans supplementing with vitamin D is approximately 50% in some countries and is an effective way to improve vitamin D status all year round [99]. Appropriate supplementation, along with a balanced and varied diet, is required for vegans and vegetarians [99, 145]. B12 supplements are recommended for vegans and vegetarians who consume small quantities of animal products as adequate B12 is not provided by plant foods. The Vegan Society UK recommends individuals take one 10 μg B12 supplement daily or take a weekly 2000 μg B12 supplement. Daily iodine supplements (150 μg) are available and are useful for individuals not consuming iodized salt or other sources of iodine in the diet (e.g., fortified foods) [133]. Kelp or other seaweed supplements are not recommended to improve iodine intake as these products have variable levels of iodine and can lead to iodine excess [146]. Individuals following a vegan or vegetarian diet must seek nutritional guidance from a health professional before considering dietary supplements.

6.2 Altering cooking, food serving, and storing practices

The cooking method used, and the way food is served and stored can influence micronutrient content [35, 115]. Using iron as an example, cooking in iron-based pans can significantly improve iron intake by transferring small quantities of iron into compound foods like sauces, soups, and stews [35, 115]. Serving iron-rich foods with foods rich in vitamin C (e.g., oranges and other fruits) can improve absorption of non-haem iron sources at each meal by facilitating conversion to Fe^{2+} [35, 115, 119]. There are various compounds that further reduce the absorption of iron, including tannins (in tea), polyphenols (in coffee), phytates (in cereals and grains), and oxalates (in spinach) [35]. These substances do not need to be avoided, however, reducing the consumption of tea and coffee during meals may help to improve iron absorption. Phytates also prevent the absorption of zinc and other divalent ions [35]. Soaking foods containing phytates can reduce the abundance of phytate and diminish their effects [35]. Other serving practices to improve micronutrient intake include spreading the intake of vitamin B12 fortified foods throughout the day to improve absorption and shaking bottles of fortified alternative milk beverages helps to mix micronutrients such as calcium that may have sunk to the bottom. A study in the US found that unshaken alternative milks had 30% less calcium than described on the label [137]. Storage can also affect the micronutrient quantity of foods with factors such as temperature and exposure to UV light being important [35, 37]. Vitamin B2 is UV sensitive and exposure to foods to sunlight can result in a significant decrease in its concentration [35].

7. Conclusions

In conclusion, vegans and vegetarians are at risk of micronutrient deficiencies. Different life stages may struggle to achieve recommendations for different micronutrients. The risk of deficiency may be more prevalent in vegan and vegetarian individuals at life stages with greater micronutrient demands. Further research into the influence of vegan and vegetarian children (0–4 years) on micronutrient nutrition is required. There are many additional factors that may affect micronutrient intake, absorption, and status at an individual level. However, all individuals following vegan and vegetarian diets, irrespective of the level of restriction chosen, should be able to achieve the RNI for all micronutrients with appropriate dietary planning, knowledge of the limitations for attaining micronutrients, and implementation of suitable precautions to improve intake, including supplementation, fortified food consumption, and implementation of other techniques to improve micronutrient bioavailability.

Acknowledgements

The Division of Food, Nutrition, and Dietetics at The University of Nottingham for backing and the BBSRC for funding. This book chapter was supported by a BBSRC doctoral training program studentship, grant number BB/M008770/1. The Vegan Society UK for the king permission to use the Vegan Eatwell Guide in this publication.

Conflict of interest

The authors declare no conflict of interest.

Author details

Elizabeth Eveleigh, Lisa Coneyworth and Simon Welham*
Division of Food, Nutrition and Dietetics, School of Biosciences, The University of Nottingham, Sutton Bonington, UK

*Address all correspondence to: simon.welham@nottingham.ac.uk

References

[1] Statista. Veganism and vegetarianism in the United Kingdom. Hamburg, Germany. 2021. Available from: https://www.statista.com/study/67944/veganism-in-the-uk/. [Accessed 19 August 2022]

[2] Phillips F. Vegetarian nutrition. Nutrition Bulletin. 2005;**30**:132-167

[3] Davis J. History of vegetarianism - Extracts from some journals 1843-48. Available from: https://ivu.org/history/vegetarian.html. [Accessed 19 August 2022]

[4] Calvert S. Ripened by human determination, 70 years of The Vegan Society. London. 2014. Available from: https://www.vegansociety.com/sites/default/files/uploads/Ripened%20by%20human%20determination.pdf. [Accessed 19 August 2022]

[5] Leitzmann C. Vegetarian nutrition: Past, present, future. The American Journal of Clinical Nutrition. 2014;**100**:496S-502S

[6] Sebastiani G, Barbero AH, Borrás-Novel C, et al. The effects of vegetarian and vegan diet during pregnancy on the health of mothers and offspring. Nutrients. 2019;**11**:557. Epub ahead of print 1 March 2019. DOI: 10.3390/nu11030557

[7] Hargreaves SM, Raposo A, Saraiva A, et al. Vegetarian diet: An overview through the perspective of quality of life domains. International Journal of Environmental Research and Public Health. 2021;**18**:4067

[8] Nezlek JB, Forestell CA. Vegetarianism as a social identity. Current Opinion in Food Science. 2020;**33**:45-51

[9] Fox N, Ward K. Health, ethics and environment: A qualitative study of vegetarian motivations. Appetite. 2008;**50**:422-429

[10] Rosenfeld DL, Burrow AL. Vegetarian on purpose: Understanding the motivations of plant-based dieters. Appetite. 2017;**116**:456-463

[11] Miki AJ, Livingston KA, Karlsen MC, et al. Using evidence mapping to examine motivations for following plant-based diets. Current Developments in Nutrition. 2020;**4**:1-15. Epub ahead of print 12 February 2020. DOI: 10.1093/CDN/NZAA013

[12] de Backer CJS, Hudders L. From meatless Mondays to meatless Sundays: Motivations for meat reduction among vegetarians and semi-vegetarians who mildly or significantly reduce their meat intake. Ecology of Food and Nutrition. 2014;**53**:639-657

[13] Kerschke-Risch P. Vegan diet: Motives, approach and duration. DOI: 10.4455/eu.2015.016

[14] Janssen M, Busch C, Rödiger M, et al. Motives of consumers following a vegan diet and their attitudes towards animal agriculture. Appetite. 2016;**105**:643-651

[15] Meatless Monday Compaigns. Meatless Monday. Available from: https://www.mondaycampaigns.org/meatless-monday. [Accessed 19 August 2022]

[16] Veganuary. Veganuary 2023. 2023. Available from: https://veganuary.com/. [Accessed 24 August 2022]

[17] MINTEL. Added value in dairy drinks, milk and cream - UK - April

2019: Attitudes towards milk, milk drinks and cream. 2019. Available from: https://reports.mintel.com/. [Accessed 7 May 2020]

[18] The Vegan Society. Business and food sales. 2022. Available from: https://www.vegansociety.com/news/media/statistics/business-and-food-sales. [Accessed 26 August 2022]

[19] Boots. Vegan supplements & vitamins. 2022. Available from: https://www.boots.com/wellness/vitaminsandsupplements/vegan-vitamins. [Accessed 26 August 2022]

[20] British Dietetic Association (BDA). British Dietetic Association confirms well-planned vegan diets can support healthy living in people of all ages. 2017. Available from: https://www.bda.uk.com/resource/british-dietetic-association-confirms-well-planned-vegan-diets-can-support-healthy-living-in-people-of-all-ages.html. [Accessed 26 August 2022]

[21] García-Morant A, Cortés-Castell E, Palazón-Bru A, et al. Macronutrients and micronutrients in spanish adult vegans (Mediterranean population). Nutrición Hospitalaria. 2020;**37**:549-558

[22] Kristensen NB, Madsen ML, Hansen TH, et al. Intake of macro- and micronutrients in Danish vegans. Nutrition Journal;**14**:1-10. Epub ahead of print 2015. DOI: 10.1186/s12937-015-0103-3

[23] Schüpbach R, Wegmüller R, Berguerand C, et al. Micronutrient status and intake in omnivores, vegetarians and vegans in Switzerland. European Journal of Nutrition. 2017;**56**:283-293

[24] Turner-McGrievy GM, Barnard ND, Scialli A, et al. Effects of a low-fat vegan diet and a Step II diet on macro- and micronutrient intakes in overweight postmenopausal women. Nutrition. 2004;**20**:738-746

[25] Eveleigh E, Coneyworth L, Zhou M, et al. Vegans and vegetarians living in Nottingham (UK) continue to be at risk of iodine deficiency. The British Journal of Nutrition. 2022:1-46

[26] Eveleigh ER, Coneyworth LJ, Avery A, et al. Vegans, vegetarians, and omnivores: How does dietary choice influence iodine intake? A systematic review. Nutrients. 2020;**12**:1606. Epub ahead of print 1 June 2020. DOI: 10.3390/nu12061606

[27] Groufh-Jacobsen S, Hess SY, Aakre I, et al. Vegans, vegetarians and pescatarians are at risk of iodine deficiency in Norway. Nutrients. 2020;**12**:1-13

[28] Fallon N, Dillon SA. Low intakes of iodine and selenium amongst vegan and vegetarian women highlight a potential nutritional vulnerability. Frontiers in Nutrition. 2020;7:72

[29] Thomas E, Nicol K, Bath SC. Iodine fortification of plant-based dairy- and fish-alternative products available in UK supermarkets. Proceedings of the Nutrition Society. 2022;**81**:E29

[30] Bath SC, Hill S, Infante HG, et al. Iodine concentration of milk-alternative drinks available in the UK in comparison with cows' milk. British Journal of Nutrition. 2017;**118**:525-532

[31] Paul AA, Kumar S, Kumar V, et al. Milk analog: Plant based alternatives to conventional milk, production, potential and health concerns. Critical Reviews in Food Science and Nutrition. 2020;**60**:3005-3023

[32] Vanga SK, Raghavan V. How well do plant based alternatives fare nutritionally

compared to cow's milk? Journal of Food Science and Technology. 2018;**55**:10-20

[33] Gilsing AMJ, Crowe FL, Lloyd-Wright Z, et al. Serum concentrations of vitamin B12 and folate in British male omnivores, vegetarians and vegans: Results from a cross-sectional analysis of the EPIC-Oxford cohort study. European Journal of Clinical Nutrition. 2010;**64**:933-939

[34] Kohlenberg-Mueller K, Raschka L. Calcium balance in young adults on a vegan and lactovegetarian diet. Journal of Bone and Mineral Metabolism. 2003;**21**:28-33

[35] Platel K, Srinivasan K. Bioavailability of micronutrients from plant foods: An update. Critical Reviews in Food Science and Nutrition. 2016;**56**:1608-1619

[36] Neufingerl N, Eilander A. Nutrient intake and status in adults consuming plant-based diets compared to meat-eaters: A systematic review. Nutrients. 2021;**14**:1-25. Epub ahead of print 1 January 2021. DOI: 10.3390/NU14010029

[37] Katamine S, Mamiya Y, Sekimoto K, et al. Differences in bioavailability of iodine among iodine-rich foods and food colors. undefined

[38] Gallagher CT, Hanley P, Lane KE. Pattern analysis of vegan eating reveals healthy and unhealthy patterns within the vegan diet. Public Health Nutrition. 2022;**25**:1310-1320

[39] Solomons NW. Plant-based diets are traditional in developing countries: 21st century challenges for better nutrition and health. Asia Pacific Journal of Clinical Nutrition. 2000;**9**(Suppl. 1):41-54. Epub ahead of print 2000. DOI: 10.1046/J.1440-6047.2000.00165.X

[40] Khandpur N, Martinez-Steele E, Sun Q. Plant-based meat and dairy substitutes as appropriate alternatives to animal-based products? The Journal of Nutrition. 2021;**151**:3-4

[41] Pointke M, Pawelzik E. Plant-based alternative products: Are they healthy alternatives? micro- and macronutrients and nutritional scoring. Nutrients. 2022;**14**:1-22. Epub ahead of print 1 February 2022. DOI: 10.3390/NU14030601

[42] Sethi S, Tyagi SK, Anurag RK. Plant-based milk alternatives an emerging segment of functional beverages: A review. Journal of Food Science and Technology. 2016;**53**:3408-3423

[43] Dineva M, Rayman MP, Bath SC. Iodine status of consumers of milk-alternative drinks versus cows' milk: Data from the UK National Diet and Nutrition Survey. British Journal of Nutrition. 2021;126:28-36. Epub ahead of print 2020. DOI: 10.1017/S0007114520003876

[44] Draper A, Lewis J, Malhotra N, et al. The energy and nutrient intakes of different types of vegetarian: A case for supplements? British Journal of Nutrition. 1993;**69**:3-19

[45] Clark CD, Bassett B, Burge MR. Effects of kelp supplementation on thyroid function in euthyroid subjects. Endocrine Practice. 2003;**9**:363-369

[46] Combet E, Ma ZF, Cousins F, et al. Low-level seaweed supplementation improves iodine status in iodine-insufficient women. British Journal of Nutrition. 2014;**112**:753-761

[47] National Institutes of Health (NIH) Office of Dietary Supplements. Iodine Fact Sheet for Consumers. 2022. Available from: https://ods.od.nih.gov/factsheets/Iodine-Consumer/. [Accessed 18 August 2022]

[48] The EAT-Lancet Commission. The planetary health diet – EAT. 2022. Available from: https://eatforum.org/eat-lancet-commission/the-planetary-health-diet-and-you/. [Accessed 24 August 2022]

[49] The British Dietetic Association (BDA). One Blue Dot Eating Patterns for Health and Environmental Sustainability. London: BDA; September 2020

[50] Shenkin A. The key role of micronutrients. Clinical Nutrition. 2006;**25**:1-13

[51] British Nutrition Foundation. Nutrition Requirements. London: British Nutrition Foundation; 2021

[52] Shenkin A. Micronutrients in health and disease. Postgraduate Medical Journal. 2006;**82**:559-567

[53] Piccoli G, Clari R, Vigotti F, et al. Vegan-vegetarian diets in pregnancy: Danger or panacea? A systematic narrative review. BJOG. 2015;**122**:623-633

[54] Kirby M, Danner E. Nutritional deficiencies in children on restricted diets. Pediatric Clinics of North America. 2009;**56**:1085-1103

[55] Ferrara P, Corsello G, Quattrocchi E, et al. Caring for infants and children following alternative dietary patterns. Journal of Pediatrics. 2017;**187**:339-340.e1

[56] Lemoine A, Giabicani E, Lockhart V, et al. Case report of nutritional rickets in an infant following a vegan diet. Archives de Pédiatrie. 2020;**27**:219-222

[57] Baldassarre ME, Panza R, Farella I, et al. Vegetarian and vegan weaning of the infant: How common and how evidence-based? A population-based survey and narrative review. International Journal of Environmental Research and Public Health. 2020;**17**:1-17

[58] Weder S, Keller M, Fischer M, et al. Intake of micronutrients and fatty acids of vegetarian, vegan, and omnivorous children (1-3 years) in Germany (VeChi Diet Study). European Journal of Nutrition. 2022;**61**:1507-1520

[59] Kiely ME. Risks and benefits of vegan and vegetarian diets in children. The Proceedings of the Nutrition Society. 2021;**80**:159-164

[60] Schürmann S, Kersting M, Alexy U. Vegetarian diets in children: A systematic review. European Journal of Nutrition. 2017;**56**:1797-1817

[61] Redecilla Ferreiro S, Moráis López A, Moreno Villares JM, et al. Position paper on vegetarian diets in infants and children. Committee on nutrition and breastfeeding of the Spanish Paediatric Association. Anales de Pediatría (English Edition). 2020;**92**:306.e1-306.e6

[62] WHO. Breastfeeding. 2022. Available from: https://www.who.int/health-topics/breastfeeding#tab=tab_1. [Accessed 26 August 2022]

[63] Karcz K, Królak-Olejnik B. Vegan or vegetarian diet and breast milk composition–a systematic review. Critical Reviews in Food Science and Nutrition. 2021;**61**:1081-1098

[64] First Steps Nutrition Trust. Eating Well: Vegan Infants and Under-5s. First Steps Nutrition Trust. London; 2020. Available from: www.firststepsnutrition.org. [Accessed 26 August 2022]

[65] Hughes J, Sanders TA. Riboflavin levels in the diet and breast milk of vegans and omnivores. The Proceedings of the Nutrition Society. 1979; 2. Available from: https://pubmed.ncbi.nlm.nih.gov/504214/ [Accessed 26 August 2022]

[66] Powers HJ. Riboflavin (vitamin B-2) and health. The American Journal of Clinical Nutrition. 2003;77:1352-1360

[67] NHS. Types of formula milk. London; 2019. Available from: https://www.nhs.uk/conditions/baby/breastfeeding-and-bottle-feeding/bottle-feeding/types-of-formula/. [Accessed 15 August 2022]

[68] Vandenplas Y, Hegar B, Munasir Z, et al. The role of soy plant-based formula supplemented with dietary fiber to support children's growth and development: An expert opinion. Nutrition. 2021;**90**:111278

[69] Lacerda Sanches V, Alves Peixoto RR, Cadore S. Phosphorus and zinc are less bioaccessible in soy-based beverages in comparison to bovine milk. Journal of Functional Foods. 2020;**65**:103728

[70] Reed MA. Considerations in planning vegan diets: Infants. Journal of the American Dietetic Association. 2001;**101**:670-676

[71] Start 4 Life. Weaning. 2022. Available from: https://www.nhs.uk/start4life/weaning/. [Accessed 26 August 2022]

[72] NHS. Vitamins for children. 2022. Available from: https://www.nhs.uk/conditions/baby/weaning-and-feeding/vitamins-for-children/. [Accessed 26 August 2022]

[73] Scientific Advisory Committee on Nutrition (SACN) & the Committee on Toxicity (COT) - Joint SACN/COT Working Group on PlantBased Drinks. SACN & COT London; 202

[74] Balasundaram P, Avulakunta ID. Human growth and development. Basics in Human Evolution. 2022:285-293

[75] Moschonis G, Papandreou D, Mavrogianni C, et al. Association of iron depletion with menstruation and dietary intake indices in pubertal girls: The healthy growth study. BioMed Research International. 2013. Epub ahead of print 2013. DOI: 10.1155/2013/423263

[76] Winzenberg T, Jones G. Vitamin D and bone health in childhood and adolescence. Calcified Tissue International. 2013;**92**:140-150

[77] Public Health England. Foods and drinks aimed at infants and young children: Evidence and opportunities for action. 2019. Available from: www.facebook.com/PublicHealthEngland. [Accessed 26 August 2022]

[78] Amit M, Cummings C, Grueger B, et al. Vegetarian diets in children and adolescents. Paediatrics & Child Health. 2010;**15**:303

[79] Desmond MA, Sobiecki JG, Jaworski M, et al. Growth, body composition, and cardiovascular and nutritional risk of 5-to 10-y-old children consuming vegetarian, vegan, or omnivore diets. American Journal of Clinical Nutrition. 2021;**113**:1565-1577

[80] Ambrosini GL, Oddy WH, Robinson M, et al. Adolescent dietary patterns are associated with lifestyle and family psycho-social factors. Public Health Nutrition. 2009;**12**:1807-1815

[81] Derbyshire E. Micronutrient intakes of British adults across mid-life: A secondary analysis of the UK National Diet and nutrition survey. Frontiers in Nutrition. 2018;**5**:1-9. Epub ahead of print 19 July 2018. DOI: 10.3389/fnut.2018.00055

[82] The Royal College of Psychiatrists, The British Dietetic Association, BEAT. Consensus statement on considerations for treating vegan patients with eating disorders

[83] Sergentanis TN, Chelmi ME, Liampas A, et al. Vegetarian diets and eating disorders in adolescents and young adults: A Systematic review. Children. 2020;**8**:12. Epub ahead of print 1 January 2021. DOI: 10.3390/CHILDREN8010012

[84] Henjum S, Brantsæter A, Kurniasari A, et al. Suboptimal iodine status and low iodine knowledge in young Norwegian women. Nutrients. 2018;**10**:941

[85] Dwyer J, Loew FM. Nutritional risks of vegan diets to women and children: Are they preventable? Journal of Agricultural and Environmental Ethics. 1994;**7**:87-109

[86] Bath SC, Rayman MP. A review of the iodine status of UK pregnant women and its implications for the offspring. Environmental Geochemistry and Health. 2015;**37**:619-629

[87] NHS. Planning your pregnancy. 2020. Available from: https://www.nhs.uk/pregnancy/trying-for-a-baby/planning-your-pregnancy/. [Accessed 26 August 2022]

[88] Milman N, Paszkowski T, Cetin I, et al. Supplementation during pregnancy: Beliefs and science. Gynecological Endocrinology. 2016;**32**:509-516

[89] NHS. Get help to buy food and milk (healthy start). 2022. Available from: https://www.healthystart.nhs.uk/. [Accessed 26 August 2022]

[90] Engel MG, Kern HJ, Brenna JT, et al. Micronutrient gaps in three commercial weight-loss diet plans. Nutrients. 2018;**10**:108. Epub ahead of print 20 January 2018. DOI: 10.3390/nu10010108

[91] Gardner CD, Kim S, Bersamin A, et al. Micronutrient quality of weight-loss diets that focus on macronutrients: results from the A to Z study. The American Journal of Clinical Nutrition. 2010;**92**:304-312

[92] von Arnim CAF, Dismar S, Ott-Renzer CS, et al. Micronutrients supplementation and nutritional status in cognitively impaired elderly persons: A two-month open label pilot study. Nutrition Journal. 2013;**12**:1-8

[93] Rémond D, Shahar DR, Gille D, et al. Understanding the gastrointestinal tract of the elderly to develop dietary solutions that prevent malnutrition. Oncotarget. 2015;**6**:13858

[94] Holland & Barrett. Vegans uncovered. 2021. Available from: https://www.hollandandbarrett.com/shop/vegan/2020-vegan-insights/. [Accessed 26 August 2022]

[95] The Nutrition Society, Lanham-New S, Gallagher A, et al. Introduction to Human Nutrition. London: Wiley; 2019. Available from: https://www.wiley.com/en-sg/Introduction+to+Human+Nutrition%2C+3rd+Edition-p-9781119476979. [Accessed 26 August 2022]

[96] Halsted CH. Absorption of water-soluble vitamins. Current Opinion in Gastroenterology. 2003;**19**:113-117

[97] Health NRC (US) C on D and Fat-Soluble Vitamins. 1989. Available from: https://www.ncbi.nlm.nih.gov/books/NBK218749/. [Accessed 26 August 2022]

[98] Bakaloudi DR, Halloran A, Rippin HL, et al. Intake and adequacy of the vegan diet. A systematic review of the evidence. Clinical Nutrition. 2021;**40**:3503-3521

[99] Weikert C, Trefflich I, Menzel J, et al. Vitamin and mineral status in a vegan diet. Deutsches Ärzteblatt International. 2020;**117**:575-582

[100] Krehl WA, Teply LJ, Sarma PS, et al. Growth-retarding effect of corn in nicotinic acid-low rations and its counteraction by tryptophane. Science. 1945;**101**:489-490

[101] Redzic S, Gupta V. Niacin deficiency. Southern Medical Journal. 2022;**45**:775

[102] Djadjo S, Bajaj T. Niacin. StatPearls. 2022. Available from: https://www.ncbi.nlm.nih.gov/books/NBK541036/. [Accessed 26 August 2022]

[103] Watanabe F, Yabuta Y, Bito T, et al. Vitamin B12-containing plant food sources for vegetarians. Nutrients. 2014;**6**:1861-1873

[104] O'Leary F, Samman S. Vitamin B12 in health and disease. Nutrients. 2010;**2**:299-316

[105] Rizzo G, Laganà AS, Rapisarda AMC, et al. Vitamin B12 among vegetarians: Status, assessment and supplementation. Nutrients; 2016;**8**:767. Epub ahead of print 29 November 2016. DOI: 10.3390/NU8120767

[106] Pawlak R, Parrott SJ, Raj S, et al. How prevalent is vitamin B12 deficiency among vegetarians? Nutrition Reviews. 2013;**71**:110-117

[107] Scott JM, Weir DG. The methyl folate trap. A physiological response in man to prevent methyl group deficiency in kwashiorkor (methionine deficiency) and an explanation for folic-acid induced exacerbation of subacute combined degeneration in pernicious anaemia. Lancet. 1981;**2**:337-340

[108] Dominguez LJ, Farruggia M, Veronese N, et al. Vitamin D sources, metabolism, and deficiency: Available compounds and guidelines for its treatment. 2021;**11**:225. Epub ahead of print 1 April 2021. DOI: 10.3390/METABO11040255

[109] Zmijewski MA. Vitamin D and human health. International Journal of Molecular Sciences; 2020;**20**:421. Epub ahead of print 1 January 2019. DOI: 10.3390/IJMS20010145

[110] Calame W, Street L, Hulshof T. Vitamin D serum levels in the UK Population, including a mathematical approach to evaluate the impact of vitamin D fortified ready-to-eat breakfast cereals: Application of the NDNS Database. Nutrients. 2020;**12**:1-14

[111] Benedik E. Sources of vitamin D for humans. International Journal for Vitamin and Nutrition Research. 2022;**92**:118-125

[112] McClements DJ. Development of next-generation nutritionally fortified plant-based milk substitutes: Structural design principles. Food;**9**. Epub ahead of print 1 April 2020. DOI: 10.3390/foods9040421

[113] Menzel J, Abraham K, Stangl GI, et al. Vegan diet and bone health—Results from the cross-sectional RBVD study. Nutrients. 2021;**13**:685

[114] Appleby P, Roddam A, Allen N, et al. Comparative fracture risk in vegetarians and nonvegetarians in EPIC-Oxford. European Journal of Clinical Nutrition. 2007;**61**:1400-1406

[115] Ems T, Lucia KS, Huecker MR. Biochemistry, Iron Absorption. StatPearls. 2022. Available from: https://www.ncbi.nlm.nih.gov/books/NBK448204/. [Accessed 26 August 2022]

[116] Waldvogel-Abramowski S, Waeber G, Gassner C, et al. Physiology of iron metabolism. Transfusion Medicine and Hemotherapy. 2014;**41**:213

[117] Micronutrients I of M (US) P on. Dietary Reference Intakes for Vitamin A, Vitamin K, Arsenic, Boron, Chromium, Copper, Iodine, Iron, Manganese, Molybdenum, Nickel, Silicon, Vanadium, and Zinc. Washington (DC): National Academies Press; 2001. Epub ahead of print 19 June 2001. DOI: 10.17226/10026

[118] Pawlak R, Berger J, Hines I. Iron status of vegetarian adults: A review of literature. American Journal of Lifestyle Medicine. 2016;**12**:486-498

[119] Henjum S, Groufh-Jacobsen S, Stea TH, et al. Iron status of vegans, vegetarians and Pescatarians in Norway. Biomolecules. 2021;**11**:1-10

[120] Ershow AG, Skeaff SA, Merkel JM, et al. Development of databases on iodine in foods and dietary supplements. Nutrients. 2018;**10**:100. Epub ahead of print 17 January. DOI: 10.3390/nu10010100

[121] Ahad F, Ganie SA. Iodine, iodine metabolism and iodine deficiency disorders revisited. Indian Journal of Endocrinology and Metabolism. 2010;**14**:13-17

[122] Fuge R. Soils and iodine deficiency. In: Essentials of Medical Geology: Revised Edition. Dordrecht: Springer Netherlands; 2013. pp. 417-432

[123] Bath SC, Button S, Rayman MP. Availability of iodised table salt in the UK - Is it likely to influence population iodine intake? Public Health Nutrition. 2014;**17**:450-454

[124] Wu T, Liu GJ, Li P, et al. Iodised salt for preventing iodine deficiency disorders. Cochrane Database of Systematic Reviews. 2002:1-20. Epub ahead of print 22 July 2002. DOI: 10.1002/14651858.cd003204

[125] de Bortoli MC, Cozzolino SMF. Zinc and selenium nutritional status in vegetarians. Biological Trace Element Research. 2009;**127**:228-233

[126] O'Kane SM, Mulhern MS, Pourshahidi LK, et al. Micronutrients, iodine status and concentrations of thyroid hormones: A systematic review. Nutrition Reviews. 2018;**76**:418-431

[127] Food Empowerment Project. Bringing Community Voices to the Table. San Jose; 2010. Available from: https://www.foodispower.org/wp-content/uploads/FEP_community_voices_report.pdf. [Accessed 30 August 2022]

[128] EUFIC. Dive into the world of vitamins and minerals. 2021. Available from: https://www.eufic.org/en/vitamins-and-minerals/article/dive-into-the-world-of-vitamins-and-minerals. [Accessed 30 August 2022]

[129] Hoffman SR, Stallings SF, Bessinger RC, et al. Differences between health and ethical vegetarians. Strength of conviction, nutrition knowledge, dietary restriction, and duration of adherence. Appetite. 2013;**65**:139-144

[130] O'Kane SM, Pourshahidi LK, Farren KM, et al. Iodine knowledge is positively associated with dietary iodine intake among women of childbearing age in the UK and Ireland. British Journal of Nutrition. 2016;**116**:1728-1735

[131] Charlton K, Yeatman H, Lucas C, et al. Poor knowledge and practices related to iodine nutrition during pregnancy and lactation in Australian women: Pre- and post-iodine fortification. Nutrients. 2012;**4**:1317-1327

[132] NHS. The eatwell guide. 2019. Available from: https://www.nhs.uk/live-well/eat-well/

food-guidelines-and-food-labels/the-eatwell-guide/. [Accessed 30 August 2022]

[133] Introducing the Vegan Eatwell Guide. 2020. Available from: https://www.bda.uk.com/resource/introducing-the-vegan-eatwell-guide.html. [Accessed 20 May 2021]

[134] WHO. Food fortification. 2022. Available from: https://www.who.int/health-topics/food-fortification#tab=tab_1. [Accessed 30 August 2022]

[135] Department of Health and Social Care. Proposal to add folic acid to flour: Consultation response. 2021. Available from: https://www.gov.uk/government/consultations/adding-folic-acid-to-flour/outcome/proposal-to-add-folic-acid-to-flour-consultation-response. [Accessed 30 August 2022]

[136] Office for Health Improvement and Disparities. Vitamin D: Call for evidence. 2022. Available from: https://www.gov.uk/government/consultations/vitamin-d-call-for-evidence/vitamin-d-call-for-evidence. [Accessed 30 August 2022]

[137] Azmina G. Vegan Savvy: The Expert's Guide to Nutrition on a Plant-based Diet. London: Pavilion Books. Available from: https://www.whsmith.co.uk/products/vegan-savvy-the-experts-guide-to-staying-healthy-on-a-plantbased-diet/azmina-govindji/paperback/9781911663416.html; 2020. [Accessed 30 August 2022]

[138] British Dietetic Association (BDA). Iodine: The debate around fortification. Available from: https://www.bda.uk.com/resource/iodine-the-debate-around-fortification.html. [Accessed 18 August 2022]

[139] Food Standards Agency (FSA). Food supplements. 2021. Available from: https://www.food.gov.uk/business-guidance/food-supplements. [Accessed 24 November 2022]

[140] British Dietetic Association (BDA). Supplements. 2022. Available from: https://www.bda.uk.com/resource/supplements.html. [Accessed 24 November 2022]

[141] Selinger E, Kühn T, Procházková M, et al. Vitamin B12 deficiency is prevalent among Czech vegans who do not use vitamin B12 supplements. Nutrients. 2019;**11**:1-800. Epub ahead of print 1 December 2019. DOI: 10.3390/NU11123019

[142] Henjum S, Brantsæter AL, Kurniasari A, et al. Suboptimal iodine status and low iodine knowledge in young Norwegian women. Nutrients. 2018;**10**:941. Epub ahead of print 21 July 2018. DOI: 10.3390/nu10070941

[143] Bailey RL, Dodd KW, Gahche JJ, et al. Best practices for dietary supplement assessment and estimation of total usual nutrient intakes in population-level research and monitoring. The Journal of Nutrition. 2019;**149**:181

[144] NHS. Vitamin D. 2020. Available from: https://www.nhs.uk/conditions/vitamins-and-minerals/vitamin-d/. [Accessed 30 August 2022]

[145] Pellinen T, Essi P, Isotalo J, et al. Replacing dietary animal-source proteins with plant-source proteins changes dietary intake and status of vitamins and minerals in healthy adults: A 12-week randomized controlled trial. European Journal of Nutrition. 2022;**3**:1391-1404. Epub ahead of print 27 November 2021. DOI: 10.1007/s00394-021-02729-3

[146] Smyth PPA, Karger S. Iodine, seaweed, and the thyroid. Basic Thyroidology/Review Article. European Thyroid Journal. 2021;**10**:101-108